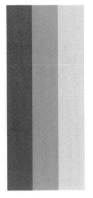

Contents

About the editors   v

List of contributors   vi

Preface   viii

Introduction   ix

1   Ageing – the biology of growing old   1
Ioan Davies

2   The demography of old age   9
Tony Warnes

3   The presentation and management of physical disease in older people   15
Sebastian Fairweather

4   The presentation and management of mental disease in older people   54
Catherine Oppenheimer

5   Prescribing and the older patient in the community   66
Michael Denham

6   Nutrition of older people   72
Helen Molyneux

7   Anticipatory care of older people in the community   80
David Beales and Alistair Tulloch

8   The practical organization of screening and socio-medical assessment in old age   89
Iain McIntosh

9   Health promotion and keeping fit in old age   95
Marion McMurdo

10   Community nursing and primary care   102
Kate Saffin

11   Institutional care of older people in the community   108
Clive Bowman

12   Disability and rehabilitation for older people   114
     Sean Brotheridge and John Young

13   Special services for older people   123
     David Lubel

14   Law and the older patient   130
     Frank Fletcher, Carlyn Leslie and Peter Scott

15   Medical ethics in community care   136
     Donald Portsmouth

16   Older people in ethnic minority groups   141
     Alistair Ritch

17   Taking the Diploma in Geriatric Medicine   147
     Bryan Moore-Smith

18   The carer's perspective   152
     Jill Pitkeathley and Carolyn Syverson

Appendix 1: The Bicester system of screening for the elderly   157

Appendix 2: McIntosh over 75s assessment questionnaire – data store   168

Appendix 3: Phoenix Surgery Anticipatory Care Model for people
             over the age of 75 years in Cirencester   174

Cardiff-Newport Questionnaire   177

Training Programme for Staywell 75+ Volunteer Visting Scheme   186

Winchester Questionnaire   187

Phoenix Surgery letters   188

Further information   191

Index   199

Community Care of Older People

Edited by

David Beales

Michael Denham

and

Alistair Tulloch

© 1998 David Beales, Michael Denham and Alistair Tulloch

Radcliffe Medical Press Ltd
18 Marcham Road, Abingdon, Oxon OX14 1AA, UK

British Library Cataloguing in Publication Data

A catalogue record for this book is available from the British Library.

ISBN 1 85775 032 2

Library of Congress Cataloging-in-Publication Data is available.

Typeset by Advance Typesetting Ltd, Oxon
Printed and bound by Redwood Books Ltd, Trowbridge, Wilts

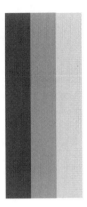

About the editors

David Beales decided to become a general practitioner after training in rheumatology and rehabilitation at Guy's and King's College Hospitals. Partnership followed in a busy South London practice and then a move to Cirencester where he combined general practice with hospital practitioner sessions in care of the elderly. He is a lead research practitioner supported by the South and West Research and Development Directorate. His particular interests are in needs assessment for disabled people and anticipatory care. He is an examiner for the Diploma in Geriatric Medicine.

Alistair Tulloch is a retired general practitioner and has been a Research Officer for the Oxford Community Health Project at the Unit of Healthcare Epidemiology, University of Oxford since 1969. He has published many papers on urgent demand, hospital discharge reports, repeat prescribing, records, disability registers, out-of-hours calls and especially on primary care of the elderly.

Michael Denham has been a consultant physician in geriatric medicine since 1973. He has written extensively on medical aspects of care and treatment of older people. He has been the Secretary and President of the British Geriatrics Society and a censor of the Royal College of Physicians of London, where he examines for the MRCP and is a past examiner for the DGM. Recently, he was chairman of the College working party which produced the report on Medication for Older People. For many years he was seconded annually to the NHS Health Advisory Service and currently he is active in several medical charities devoted to the care of older people.

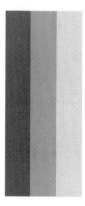

List of contributors

Dr David Beales MB, BS, MRCP (UK), MRCS,
   LRCP, MRCGP, DCH, Dobst, RCOG
General Practitioner
Phoenix Surgery
9 Chesterton Lane
Cirencester
Gloucestershire GL7 1XG

Dr Clive Bowman BSc(Hons), MB, FRCP
Consultant Geratologist
Weston General Hospital
Grange Road
Weston-super-Mare
Avon BS23 4TQ

Dr Sean Brotheridge MB, MRCP
Senior Registrar
Department of Healthcare for the Elderly
St Luke's Hospital
Bradford BD5 0NN

Dr Ioan Davies BSc, PhD
Lecturer in Biological Gerontology
Department of Cell and Structural Biology
University of Manchester Medical School
Oxford Road
Manchester M13 9PT

Dr Michael Denham MA, MD, FRCP
Consultant Geriatrician
Northwick Park Hospital
Watford Road
Harrow HA1 3UJ

Dr Sebastian Fairweather MA, PhD, FRCP
Consultant Physician
Department of Clinical Geratology
Radcliffe Infirmary
Oxford OX2 6HE

Frank Fletcher LLB, NP
Solicitor
Bird Semple
249 West George Street
Glasgow G2 4RB

Carlyn Leslie BSc, MB, ChB, MRCP
Department of Medicine for the Elderly
Stobhill NHS Trust
Balomock Road
Glasgow G21 3UW

Dr David Lubel MB, MRCP
Consultant Geriatrician
Northwick Park Hospital
Watford Road
Harrow HA1 3UJ

Dr Iain McIntosh BA, MB, ChB, Dobst,
   RCOG, DGM, RCP
11 Shirras Brae
St Ninians
Stirling FK7 0AY

Professor Marion McMurdo MD, MRCP
Professor of Ageing and Health
Department of Medicine
University of Dundee
Ninewells Hospital and Medical School
Dundee DD1 9SY

Helen Molyneux MSc, BSc(Hons), SRD
Senior Dietitian
Regional Rehabilitation Unit
Northwick Park Hospital
Watford Road
Harrow HA1 3UJ

Dr Bryan Moore-Smith MA, BM.BCh, FRCP
Consultant Geriatrician
The Ipswich Hospital
Heath Road
Ipswich
Suffolk IP4 5PD

Dr Catherine Oppenheimer BM, FRCP
Consultant Psychiatrist
Department of Psychiatry
  and Old Age
The Warneford Hospital
Headington
Oxford OX3 7JX

Baroness Jill Pitkeathley OBE, BA (Econ)
Chief Executive
Carers National Association
Ruth Pitter House
20–25 Glasshouse Yard
London EC1A 4JS

Dr Donald Portsmouth MA, MB, FRCP, FRCP(E),
  DTM&H
Senior Clinical Lecturer and Honorary
  Consultant in Geriatrics
Department of Biomedical Science
  and Ethics
University of Birmingham
Birmingham B15 2TT

Dr Alistair Ritch MB, FRCP, FRCP(E)
Consultant Geriatrician
Department of Geriatric Medicine
City Hospital
Dudley Road
Birmingham B18 7QH

Kate Saffin MPhil, RGN, RHV
Unit of Health Care – Epidemiology
Institute of Health Sciences
University of Oxford, Old Road
Oxford OX3 7LF

Dr Peter Scott BSc, MD, FRCP(G)
Clinical Director
Department of Medicine for the Elderly
Stobhill NHS Trust
Balomock Road
Glasgow G21 3UW

Carolyn Syverson BA
Primary Care Development Officer
Carers National Association
Ruth Pitter House
20–25 Glasshouse Yard
London EC1A 4JS

Dr Alistair Tulloch MD, FRCGP, Dobst, RCOG
36 Church Lane
Wendlebury
Oxon OX6 8PN

Professor Tony Warnes BSc, PhD
Centre for Ageing and Rehabilitation Studies
University of Sheffield
Northern General Hospital
Herries Road
Sheffield S5 7AU

Dr John Young MSc, MB, BS, FRCP
Consultant Geriatrician
St Luke's Hospital
Little Horton Lane
Bradford BD5 0NA

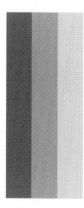

Preface

No one is so old that he does not think he could live another year

Cicero, De Senectute, c.44 BC

Who would not want to 'live another day' if that day were free from persistent disability and if pleasure in living were preserved? It is well recognized that many older people can enjoy good health, run their own household, play useful roles with their children, grandchildren, even great grandchildren and play a prominent role in community affairs. Indeed, older people represent an enormous human resource of knowledge, experience and expertise.

The aim of the majority of older people is to remain in good health. To help them achieve this requires enthusiasm, basic knowledge and effective teamwork from all health professionals involved in their care.

This book provides those interested in the overall care of older people with much relevant information. The editors hope that readers will also be stimulated by a desire to learn more and respond to the challenge of maintaining others' good health into old age.

David Beales
Michael Denham
Alistair Tulloch
October 1997

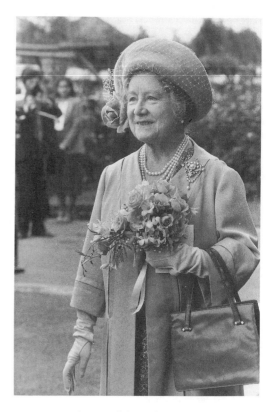

Photograph by Richard Slade

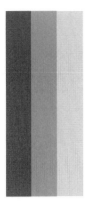

Introduction

The management and organization of care underwent fundamental change with the new contract in 1990, which required radical changes in the care of people aged 75 years or more. The new system was untested and general practitioners were untrained in and unconvinced of the merits of certain elements of the work, with the result that the implementation of the programme has been patchy and in some instances poor.

This new and up-to-date textbook reviews the case for and against anticipatory care, helping doctors to form an objective view on the subject. The section on care in general practice also offers advice on the organization of a programme to meet the requirements for socio-medical assessment under the 1990 contract for which the primary care team is ill-prepared and on which it was given no guidelines by the Government. Dr McIntosh, whose system is probably the most widely used in Scotland, has contributed a special section on this subject and appendices are included on the system used by Dr Beales and Dr Tulloch in their practices. It is hoped that general practitioners will find these helpful and use them partly or wholly in the organization of their own programmes.

In the past 20 years it has been recognized that care in this field should be directed equally towards the control of suffering and the maintenance of function to enable older people to remain independent for as long as possible in their chosen setting, able to pursue their remaining aspirations and to lead the best life possible. Treatment of disease, of course, remains the bedrock of our work but it must be coupled with good standards of rehabilitation and prosthetic support to maintain patient function. This can only be achieved by effective teamwork within the primary care team and in close co-operation with public health and hospital staff to provide high standards of patient assessment as well as social services. The diverse authorship of this book emphasizes the need for integrated multi-disciplinary care and includes contributions from the perspective of patients and carers.

The book also addresses all the important dimensions of community care of older people. In many areas, of course, medical care in old age is similar to that in younger people. Thus the chapter by Dr Fairweather concentrates on the manner in which disorders present and are managed differently in old age. In this section certain problems of particular importance in old age, e.g. recurrent falls are given particular attention.

With an emphasis on the evaluation and organization of socio-medical assessment in old age this book is very useful to all doctors in general practice or preparing for general practice, especially if they are taking the Diploma in Geriatric Medicine. It is equally useful for nurses, health visitors, social workers and others involved in this field, e.g. all care workers in nursing homes.

Community Care of Older People is neither too concise nor a bulky work of reference, but occupies the middle ground, where the most useful textbooks for general practice are usually to be found.

CHAPTER 1

Ageing – the biology of growing old

Ioan Davies

This chapter introduces the biology of growing old. Changes in physiological effectiveness with increasing age are discussed, and the scope for modifying these changes is examined, with a view to improving the quality of life in later years. Finally, some of the mechanisms of ageing are discussed.

What is ageing?

All organisms undergo a period of development and growth before they become reproductively mature. Under natural conditions, the time of reproductive activity in most species is short, and is followed closely by death. In the wild, ageing is probably not a major determinant of the time of death. Most of the recognizable features of ageing occur in animals protected from their environment, e.g. humans and domestic species, and after the period of reproductive activity has ceased. The definition of ageing (Box 1.1)

Box 1.1: Definitions

> *Ageing* the period of the lifespan characterized by a *failure to maintain homeostasis* under conditions of physiological stress. This failure is associated with a decrease in viability and an increase in vulnerability of the individual
>
> *Longevity* Maximum lifespan recorded for a species

implies that ageing is in the later part of the lifespan. However, events that obviously take place during the early development of complex multicellular organisms, such as mammals, influence ageing to a great extent. Notice that particular emphasis is placed upon the *failure to maintain homeostasis* because it is in the integration of complex physiological functions that the greatest age-associated changes are observed.[1] There is one certainty, and that is longevity is defined by a specific endpoint – death, which enables us to define accurately the length of the lifespan.

There are a number of predictions for the maximum length of life of the human species. Olshansky[2] has reviewed the current evidence and argues that as the actuarial estimate of average life expectancy approaches 80 years, large reductions in the death rate are required to produce even marginal increases in mean lifespan. Some demographers have estimated that life expectancy will soon approach 100 years but these estimates are based on unrealistic changes in human behaviour and mortality patterns. However, even though Olshansky[2] claims that there is no indication that humans can have a maximum lifespan much greater than 110 years, a Frenchwoman, Jeanne Calment recently died at the age of 122 years. This is a milestone in the survival of humankind and fuels the belief that breakthroughs in molecular and cellular biology will permit the extension of the average, and ultimately our maximum lifespan. It is also clear that unless there is a parallel reduction in the disabling diseases of later life, by a simultaneous compression of morbidity, the quality of our pro-longed existence may be poor.

Age-associated changes in physiological effectiveness

As we get older the body composition changes; lean body mass is reduced and the fat content of the body increases.[3] Among other things this can alter the pharmacodynamics of fat-soluble drugs. The location of body fat also changes with age; a general loss of fat from beneath the skin is associated with an increase in the trunk region. In addition, water is lost progressively from the body, and is redistributed within the body compartments. This in turn alters the pharmaco-dynamics of water-soluble therapeutic agents.

The skin, particularly those areas exposed to the sun, usually shows marked age-associated changes.[4] Wrinkles, and other blemishes, are caused by alterations that occur in the cells of the skin, the subcutaneous fat and the connective tissues. Age-changes in connective tissues take place despite the damage done by prolonged exposure to ultraviolet (UV) radiation, which is a major factor in skin cancer.

The musculoskeletal system

Bone is a living tissue and constantly undergoes remodelling in response to forces applied to it during exercise, and after damage. Bone loss in ageing is universal, but occurs at different rates in individuals. Bone loss is seen in everyone by the fifth decade, in both sexes, and the rate of loss is greater in females after the menopause.

Osteoporosis

This condition is not one entity but the result of several age-associated events, all leading to a reduction in bone mass. Osteoporosis has characteristic features that separate it from other forms of bone disease. In simple terms, a person with osteoporosis has a lower bone mass than might be expected from age and sex norms, and an increased risk of fracture. A major factor in the determination of bone density (see Box 1.2) in old age is the bone mass at maturity. The differences in bone mass between the sexes with age may be accounted for by the lower bone

Box 1.2: Determinants of bone density

- Gender
- Genetic background
- Endocrinology
- Nutrition
- Ethnicity
- Exercise
- Age

densities at maturity and more rapid bone loss after the menopause. Given that osteoporosis is only apparent at some critical bone mass, this level will be reached sooner in people starting with lower bone densities. Clearly, if women at the age of 18 years have a 20% lower bone mass than men of the same age, a more rapid bone loss in women aged over 50 years might account for the higher prevalence of osteoporosis in women, suggesting some critical level of bone mass beyond which there is an associated risk of fracture. The rate of bone loss in women is often described as linear after the age of 50. However, it is now known that the rate of bone loss is most rapid in the 5–10 years after the menopause.

In younger adults (20–50 years of age) bone fracture is usually by violent direct trauma to the bone, whereas in old people the fractures result from moderate to minimal trauma. In old people, the sites of fractures are often different, taking place through the trabecular region close to the joint. The trauma that precipitates an osteoporotic fracture is nearly always a fall (see Box 1.3). However, with vertebral collapse fractures there may be no history of trauma, or the force causing the collapse may be muscular.

Cartilage

Age also affects cartilaginous structures. In old people the joint cartilage tends to become thinner, due in part to wear and tear. Furthermore, cartilage can become calcified with age making flexible joints like the costal cartilage more rigid, affecting movements of the rib cage during breathing. The fibrocartilage of the intervertebral

Box 1.3: Ageing changes and functional consequences

Type of change	Functional alteration
Age-associated changes	• Diminished postural control • Abnormal gait • Weakness • Poor vision • Slow reaction time
Specific disease	• Arthritis • Cerebrovascular disease • Parkinson's disease • Cataract • Retinal degeneration • Menière's disease • Blackouts (large number of causative factors involved: low blood sugar, low blood pressure, disturbances in heart rhythm, acute onset of a stroke, epilepsy, etc.)
Drugs	• Sedatives • Blood pressure lowering agents • Antidiabetic drugs • Alcohol
Environmental factors	• Slippery surfaces (particularly street surfaces in bad weather; contributing factors may include poor footwear and walking appliances) • Uneven surfaces • Tripping over unseen obstacles

discs loses water leading to a reduced ability to bear weight.

Muscle

Changes in muscle function are another feature of advanced age. However, it is very difficult to differentiate between a loss of function due to inactivity and a genuine age-associated change.[5] In skeletal muscle there is a general reduction in muscle mass with increasing age, partly due to cell death and partly atrophic change. Atrophy is most likely due to inactivity.

In conjunction with a loss of muscle mass, there is an overall reduction in muscle strength. Fast-twitch fibres appear to atrophy before slow-twitch muscles. Thus, *strength* appears to be influenced more than *endurance* in old people, but it is known that people in their 70s can increase their muscle strength using suitable training programmes.

There is now extensive research into the reversal of the effects of muscle atrophy with age. Injection of natural growth hormone (GH) (see later) is able to promote muscle growth in old people and the use of such compounds may make it possible to regain sufficient muscle function to undergo rehabilitation. Advances in the use of artificial electrical stimulation to muscles in chronically disabled people are also proceeding rapidly.

The cardiovascular system

One of the biggest problems we have in understanding the effect of age on the heart is the impact of disease on the heart itself.[6] About 75% of men have significant narrowing of the coronary arteries by the age of 60 years. In women this figure is about 25% (at the same age), although by 80 years of age about 60% of women have similar damage. However, in old people without coronary artery disease cardiac output is *not* markedly affected by age. There are age-changes in the blood vessels. They become less compliant because of changes in the connective tissue components of the vessel wall. This means that a greater pressure has to be exerted by the heart to pump blood through the vessels. This leads to a rise in systolic blood pressure that increases the workload on the heart. It is typical to find old, healthy elderly people with a mild left ventricular hypertrophy to handle this extra work.

There is considerable evidence to show that old people benefit by carrying out regular physical exercise. Old people can increase their maximum oxygen consumption by carrying out programmes of endurance exercise such as walking, cycling or jogging. This can improve cardiac output and increase blood flow and oxygen to the skeletal muscles. However, it is important that middle-aged and elderly people have a thorough medical examination before embarking on such an exercise regimen.

Atheroma that reduces the size of blood vessels with age is another age-associated change that can be influenced by diet and exercise. The blood levels of fats tend to increase with age and this is related to both diet and amount of exercise taken.

The nervous system

The functional implications of age-related changes in the structure and function of the CNS are immense. The weight and volume of the human brain declines by about 10% between 30 and 90 years of age due to a progressive loss of neocortical neurones with age but the scale of the losses is not thought to be as great as previously. The cerebellum loses approximately 25% of the Purkinje neurones, which are involved in movement coordination, perhaps explaining changes in gait and balance in older people.

Neurones in the cerebral cortex are capable of re-growing their connections with other neurones and such neurones from old people (with no previous evidence of memory disorder, or other brain damage) have greater numbers of connections than normal young adults. Thus, there is the possibility of repair and reconstruction as long as there is no brain disease. In Alzheimer's disease

there is a significant loss of neurones, and a significant reduction in the number of interneuronal connections.

The speed of conduction of a nerve impulse decreases with age. There is also an increase in the amount of the age-pigment, lipofuscin, in neurones with age. It is usual to find the occasional neurofibrillary tangle (NFT) and senile plaque in aged brains, although these structures are commonly associated with Alzheimer's disease and senile dementia. The NFT represents damage to the neurone itself and leads to the alteration of its internal structure. The senile plaques appear to be the sites of the breakdown of neurones, which in turn are being cleared up by local glial cells.

Age-associated changes in neurotransmitter chemicals of the nervous system may be responsible for the failure to integrate functions properly in old age. Levels of noradrenaline increase dramatically in old people and may be involved in an age-associated increase in blood pressure. Levels of acetylcholine in the brain are thought to be reduced with age, and this has a negative influence on memory function.

Our view of the aged brain has changed dramatically over the past 20 years. The finding of a continued ability to grow connections to other neurones in older people has triggered an interest in newly discovered growth factors which may be able to help the brain recover function more rapidly.

The special senses

Age-associated deterioration of the special senses is a major cause of disability in elderly people.[7,8]

Eye

Typical age-associated changes in the eye include slight shrinkage of the eyeball to produce long-sightedness, and alterations to the proteins of the cornea and the lens making them more likely to scatter light. The curvature of the cornea changes making astigmatism more common in the elderly. The lens also 'hardens' making it more difficult to focus light effectively. Loss of nerve cells from the retina might take place and metabolic changes in the retinal pigment epithelium could predispose to damage. The vitreous humor, which is partially composed of connective tissues, undergoes some deterioration which may eventually lead to a detachment of the retina. Consequently, old people usually need brighter conditions in order to be able to see well, although very bright lights can lead to problems of 'dazzle'.

Ear

In the ear, degeneration of nerve cells can lead to a reduction in sensitivity to sound, and there are also reports of a loss of nerve fibres in the nerve involved in balance and equilibrium.

Taste and smell

An age-associated decline in taste and smell is not well understood. However, some old people complain of being unable to taste food, or even to detect when they feel thirsty, which leads to significant problems in other aspects of homeostasis.

Control of body systems – homeostasis

Much of the preceding discussion suggests that the body has considerable reserves that enable it to reach advanced old age (say more than 75 years) with many faculties unchanged. In the 'definition' of ageing (see Box 1.1) the key term *maintaining homeostasis under conditions of physiological stress* was emphasized; although old people vary considerably in their abilities to regulate their body functions.

Temperature regulation is frequently used as an example of an age-associated decline in homeostasis. There is an age-associated reduction in the regulation of body temperature.[9] Even fit and healthy old people appear to have substantial deficits in temperature detection. Old people fail to discriminate temperature differences: young people can distinguish about 1 °C, while many old people find it difficult to discriminate 4 °C. Therefore, there is a need not only for public awareness of the problem, but to improve self-awareness of the defect.

What biological explanation is there for this deterioration? Temperature perception occurs in the skin and research has shown that cold receptors are highly dependent on a good oxygen supply, which can decrease in the skin in old age. Other skin changes, such as thinning and

wrinkling, can also affect the operation of temperature receptors, while alterations in vasomotor autonomic regulation reduce the efficiency of blood flow in the skin. The reduced body water of a frail elderly person also predisposes them to rapid changes in temperature.

Advances in the treatment of age-associated change

The endocrine system regulates homeostasis in multicellular organisms. The latter part of the lifespan is associated with a decline in homeostasis, arguing a case for an age-related decline in endocrine function, leading to alterations in, for example, mineral, glucose, water and electrolyte metabolism.

There is evidence from work with GH that manipulation of the endocrine milieu can influence some aspects of age-associated change. For example, muscle tissue from aged men can respond to GH stimulation by increasing in mass, although to the author's knowledge, strength has not been assessed. There is also circumstantial evidence that neurotransmitters and neuroendocrine factors regulating anterior pituitary hormone secretion are intimately involved in ageing. Administration of drugs that increase hypothalamic noradrenaline and dopamine activity can delay, or reverse these events.[10]

Mechanisms and theories of ageing

A successful theory of ageing must explain a decline in the functional ability of older organisms. Therefore it must explain the cellular and molecular events that result in a breakdown of cellular function and presumably cause the physiological deterioration described above. However, there are bigger questions. Why do we have to die? This question is probably as old as the sentient human species and recently an evolutionary theory has been put forward to explain why we might have a determinate lifespan (see below). The ideas about how and why we age can be divided into two groups (see Box 1.4).[1] The first concerns possible genetic mechanisms that could cause ageing. The second group deals with a series of random events that could explain age-effects (stochastic mechanisms).

Box 1.4: Mechanisms of ageing

• **Genetic mechanisms**	• Evolution
	• Programmes
• **Stochastic mechanisms**	• Genomic theories
	• Errors in protein synthesis
	• Free radicals

The evolution of ageing

Most of the genetic theories about ageing revolve around the time it takes to reproduce and produce the first offspring. It has been argued that ageing is a beneficial, or adaptive, mechanism that enables the removal of the less reproductively able at the end of the lifespan. An implication of this theory is that some special mechanism is encoded in the genome the purpose of which is to end life. However, survival data do not support the idea of programmed ageing. For example, deaths do not increase sharply at any particular stage of the lifespan as might be expected if a death mechanism was suddenly being switched on. It is also difficult to envisage how a programme would be selected for during evolution because of the high, random mortality in the early part of the natural lifespan. Further, natural selection is least effective in manipulating characteristics expressed late in life.

More recently, evolutionary theory has suggested an explanation for the observed limitation in lifespan. The disposable soma theory[11] attempts to explain mortality based on the allocation of resources to individual, and ultimately, to species survival. However, although the theory gives a rationale for the evolution of a determinate lifespan, it has yet to provide a specific physiological mechanism. It is also not clear why imperfect proteins, which are thought to cause senescence should be the source of deterioration and ageing of cells and organisms under natural conditions. More likely, in a natural environment it is the maintenance of coordinated homeostatic mechanisms, in the face of extreme environmental perturbations, that determines overall survival.

Genome-based theories

DNA has been considered the prime target for the cause of ageing. Damaged DNA as an explanation

of ageing is attractive, particularly if ageing reduces an ability to repair such damage, leading to an accumulation of defects. DNA is susceptible to damage by a variety of internal or external events (see Box 1.5). However, the effect of damage would depend on two key factors:

• not all DNA is transcribed in differentiated cells, including the non-dividing cells of the central nervous system and skeletal muscle

• probably the most vulnerable cells to these forms of damage are mitotic cells.

Damage to chromosomes and DNA has been the subject of much research, but the outcome is that there is no clear relationship between DNA damage and ageing, and no convincing evidence of a decline in DNA repair with age.

Box 1.5: Sources of DNA damage

Internal	**External**
Free radicals	Radiation
	• UV light
Temperature	• γ-rays
	• X-rays
	Chemicals
	Viruses

Non-genomic theories about ageing

Ageing can be explained as random structural or chemical damage to cells. Many of these theories are probably only of historical interest, such as the waste product, rate of living and errors in protein synthesis theory. It is now doubted whether errors in protein synthesis are a primary mechanism in ageing. However, inactive proteins do increase in aged cells and tissues.

Proteins in aged cells undergo post-translational modifications. For example, the red blood cell (RBC) makes an interesting model for the ageing of protein macromolecules. RBCs have a lifespan of about 120 days and as they get older several enzymes have been shown to accumulate in inactive or abnormal forms. The RBC does not contain a nucleus and protein synthesis is not taking place when these abnormalities are detected. Thus, these abnormal proteins must be due to modifications taking place after protein synthesis.

One of the major current mechanisms is the free-radical theory.[12] Free radicals are formed by the splitting of a covalent bond in a molecule so that each atom joined by the bond retains an electron from the shared pair. These reactions are common in normal cell physiology, and free radicals are required to drive the equilibrium of normal oxygen metabolism in mitochondria. Normally, these highly reactive chemicals are under rigid control. A well-described battery of chemical defences guards against the escape of free radicals into the cell. However, uncontrolled free-radical reactions have been proposed as an important cause of cellular pathology, and as a primary event in ageing. Free-radical damage is thought to take place throughout the lifespan causing a progressive deterioration of both nuclear and cytoplasmic components, the mitochondrion being a prime target.

The cell is protected against free-radical damage by several mechanisms. A peptide, glutathione, protects against the toxic effects of oxygen. Hydrogen peroxide can be removed by enzymes such as catalases and peroxidases, while superoxide dismutase specifically removes the superoxide radical. Several 'scavenging' systems are also present to protect the cell from lipid peroxides. Vitamin E is incorporated into membrane structure and may trap free radicals. There are age-associated reductions in glutathione, glutathione reductase and superoxide dismutase in some tissues, but no correlation has been found between the maximum lifespan potential and levels of superoxide dismutase in primates. Thus, no linkage has been found yet between the length of lifespan and the level of protective antioxidant mechanisms in an organism. Attempts to extend animal survival by feeding antioxidants throughout the lifespan have been inconclusive but results in these animals are difficult to interpret.

'Pacemaker' theories

The theories described above are directed at the explanation of molecular and cellular changes that may cause ageing in multicellular organisms. If any of the events described above took place then cellular dysfunction would be observed. If the deterioration occurred in many cells, in many organs, the system would become inefficient and ultimately 'age'. However, several theories have implicated 'organ systems' as a cause of ageing, the most notable being the immune and neuroendocrine systems.

Certain fundamental changes occur in molecules with time, e.g. thermodynamic alterations. However, while these modifications take place at a given rate, they may be modified by other external factors, including alterations in the internal environment regulated by the endocrine system. It is possible that the endocrine system acts as a 'pacemaker' for ageing in multicellular organisms. For example, the rate of accumulation of DNA damage could be influenced by hormonal events that accelerate or retard repair.

Conclusion

Physical and functional deterioration occur with ageing. The neuroendocrine system may be a major factor in this age-associated failure in homeostasis. The maintenance of life relies on correct gene expression. To function appropriately, the organism also has to integrate gene expression in many systems simultaneously. Although neuroendocrine and endocrine effects may not be the primary cause of the age-associated decline in function, they may modify certain associated phenomena. The effect of endocrine stimulation is to alter gene expression directly in target tissues, and indirectly in other organs. The evidence discussed above suggests that endocrine manipulation can restore some aspects of regulation of essential processes.

The introduction of therapeutic measures designed to re-establish homeostatic control may slow the rate of deterioration in older organisms leading to modification of the effects of advancing age and improving the quality of life of the elderly. However, if current ideas about the cellular and molecular mechanisms of ageing are correct, then the effects of these manipulations can only be temporary.

References

1 Davies I (1992) Aging and the endocrine system, in *Textbook of Geriatric Medicine and Gerontology* (eds Brocklehurst JC, Tallis RC, Fillit HM), 4th edn. Churchill Livingstone, Edinburgh.

2 Olshansky SJ, Carnes BA and Cassel CK (1993) The aging of the human species. *Scientific American*, **268(April)**:18–24.

3 Lye M (1992) Disturbances of homeostasis, in *Textbook of Geriatric Medicine and Gerontology* (eds Brocklehurst JC, Tallis RC, Fillit HM), 4th edn. Churchill Livingstone, Edinburgh.

4 Dalziel KL and Bickers DR (1992) Skin aging, in *Textbook of Geriatric Medicine and Gerontology* (eds Brocklehurst JC, Tallis RC, Fillit HM), 4th edn. Churchill Livingstone, Edinburgh.

5 Goldberg AP and Hagberg JM (1990) Physical exercise in the elderly, in *Handbook of the Biology of Aging* (eds Schneider EL, Rowe JW), 3rd edn. Academic Press Inc., San Diego.

6 Lakatta EG (1990) Heart and circulation, in *Handbook of the Biology of Aging* (eds Schneider EL, Rowe JW), 3rd edn. Academic Press Inc., San Diego.

7 Brodie SE (1992) Aging and disorders of the eye, in *Textbook of Geriatric Medicine and Gerontology* (eds Brocklehurst JC, Tallis RC, Fillit HM), 4th edn. Churchill Livingstone, Edinburgh.

8 Fisch L and Brooks DN (1992) Disorders of hearing, in *Textbook of Geriatric Medicine and Gerontology* (eds Brocklehurst JC, Tallis RC, Fillit HM), 4th edn. Churchill Livingstone, Edinburgh.

9 Wollner L and Collins KJ (1992) Disorders of the autonomic system, in *Textbook of Geriatric Medicine and Gerontology* (eds Brocklehurst JC, Tallis RC, Fillit HM), 4th edn. Churchill Livingstone, Edinburgh.

10 Meites J (1988) Neuroendocrine biomarkers of aging in the rat. *Experimental Gerontology* **23**:349–58.

11 Kirkwood TBL (1995) The evolution of aging. *Reviews in Clinical Gerontology* **5**:3–9.

12 Gutteridge JMC (1994) Free radicals and aging. *Reviews in Clinical Gerontology* **4**:279–88.

CHAPTER 2

The demography of old age

Tony Warnes

Demography and population ageing

Demography is the study of the size and structure of human populations. It has mainly been concerned with the rates of births and deaths and the ages at which they occur. Fertility, migration and mortality determine the rate of growth or decline of a population and its age structure.

In pre-industrial Europe, and in some of the poorest countries of the world today, both fertility and mortality rates were and are very high. Each female gives birth to many children during her reproductive years, but relatively few babies survive beyond one year of age, and even among older children and young adults (especially mothers), mortality rates are much higher than in the affluent world today. Average life expectancy from birth can be as low as 30 years and has rarely been more than 40 years. The result is a population with a very young age structure. In Bangladesh, more than 40% of the population are less than 16 years of age and only 3% are at least 65 years of age.

The UK has a very different demographic structure. The major change began in several north-west European countries during the second half of the nineteenth century. Rates of mortality decreased, more infants survived and family sizes increased. Some decades later a rapid fall in fertility began. There have been reverses (as with high mortality rates during major wars and high birth rates after them) and long pauses too, but by the present day, in virtually the whole of Europe, north America, Australasia and Japan, a 'demographic transition' to unprecedentedly low fertility and mortality has been completed. Each female gives birth to few children during her life (rarely more than three). Very few babies die as infants, and mortality rates up to 50 years of age are exceedingly low. Average life expectancy has increased to at least 70 years of age. The result is an age structure with relatively few children and a high share of older people – usually more than one-fifth are at least 60 years of age. In the UK in 1994, 19.5% of the population were aged less than 15 years and more than 15% at least 65 years.

Perceptions and realities of ageing

Even these basic facts challenge some frequently-heard generalizations about Britain's 'ageing population'. It is first realized that the country's age structure has been changing throughout this century and that the highest growth rates of the older population were during the 1930s and 1940s (Table 2.1). For a century, even through decades of economic depression and immense war efforts, our societies have adjusted to an increased absolute and relative number of older people. Living and health standards have improved, while the contribution of older people to production has reduced through the spread of retirement. But earlier retirement, like shorter working hours, longer holidays, longer schooling and extended higher education and training, is a mark of a more productive and leisured labour force and economy.

Second is the realization that the dominant influence on age structure is the level of fertility – both

Table 2.1: The number of elderly people by age in Great Britain, 1901–91

Year	Population (× 1000)				Share of total (%)			Annual growth (%)*		
	60+	70+	80+	All ages	60+	70+	80+	60+	70+	80+
1911	3434	1298	251	42 082	8.2	3.1	0.6	1.8	2.0	1.4
1931	5314	1962	376	46 038	11.5	4.3	0.8	2.2	2.1	2.0
1951	7890	3399	730	50 225	15.7	6.8	1.5	2.0	2.8	3.4
1971	10 512	4599	1263	55 515	18.9	8.3	2.3	1.6	1.5	2.2
1991	11 731	6174	1824	56 388	20.8	10.9	3.2	0.6	1.3	2.1

*Average annual growth rate in previous decade, except for 1951 which is since 1931.
Source: Falconer P and Rose LR (1991) *Older Britons: a survey.* University of Strathclyde, Glasgow, Table 1.2; Central Statistical Office (1994) *Annual Abstract of Statistics (1994).* HMSO, London, Table 2.5.

Table 2.2: Live births in England and Wales, 1911–90

Birth decade	Births (× 1000)	Change on prior decade (%)	Decade reach age 60+	Decade reach age 80+
1911–20	8096		1970s	1990s
1921–30	7127	−12.0	1980s	2000s
1931–40	6065	−14.9	1990s	2010s
1941–50	7251	+19.6	2000s	2020s
1951–60	7075	−2.4	2010s	2030s
1961–70	8326	+17.7	2020s	2040s
1971–80	6472	−22.3	2030s	2050s
1981–90	6613	+2.2	2040s	2060s

Source: OPCS (1987) *Birth Statistics: Historical Series of Statistics from Registrations of Births in England and Wales, 1837–1983.* OPCS (1991) *Population Trends,* **66**, Table 9.

now and in the recent past. The absolute number of people reaching the threshold of old age during a decade is determined first by the number born 60 years ago, and second by survival (net migration is generally least important). The relative share of the population that elderly people will form in future decades is dependent upon the birth rate. Just because the circumstances that would restore fertility to the level of the 1960s cannot be envisaged, this does not mean that it will not happen. Below-replacement fertility can be viewed as analogous to exceptionally high unemployment, making it easier to anticipate that the phase might pass.

The numbers born in successive decades have fluctuated intricately during this century. A substantial reduction in births during the 1920s and 1930s was followed by a one-fifth increase during the 1940s (Table 2.2). After a pause during the 1950s, there was a further substantial increase in births during the 1960s. This was followed by a 22% fall during the 1970s, and a minor recovery during the 1980s. The consequence is that there will be substantial increases in the number who reach their 60s during the first

and third decades of the next century, and a substantial drop in the 2030s. Similarly, the number of people reaching their 80s is likely to increase in the 2020s and 2040s, and fall sharply in the 2050s. This is not a prospect of ever-mounting numbers in old age.

Why then do alarmist representations of the changes in our age structure have such widespread currency? Their foundation is less in demography than in public sector finances and political ideologies. There are particular concerns about the cost of government expenditure on old-age income support and health and social care, and a spreading lobby for the state's contribution to be reduced. Later chapters will explain some of the reasons for the increasing use of health services by older people (but it is worth noting that the demands of children and younger adults are increasing faster).

The other important demographic component of the scenario for mounting numbers of older people and mounting health care demands from them, is recent and prospective trends in late-age mortality and morbidity.

Late-age mortality trends and population projections

The principal reason for the rise in mean life expectancy at birth in England and Wales from 50 years in 1901 to around 80 years in 1992 has been an enormous decrease in infant mortality. By 1992, the England and Wales annual death rate for infants under one year was 6.5 per 1000, only 4.7% of the figure during 1901–05 (Table 2.3). Death rates during later working life and the retirement years have fallen less, e.g. the annual death rate at 75–84 years during 1971–75 was 88 per 1000, nearly 70% of the level in the early 1900s.

Improvements have been accelerating, at first gently but by the 1980s at 2.6% a year. By 1992, the 75–84 years death rate was 69.2, just over one half of the level at the start of the century. The growth rates shown in Table 2.3 show that mortality rates in early retirement and at the oldest ages have also fallen increasingly rapidly in recent decades, but that the annual reduction of the infant mortality rate (4.7%) is higher than ever before. It therefore remains the case that reductions in infant mortality are a major reason for the ageing of the population.

The absolute and relative size of the future elderly population cannot be predicted precisely. While official population projections are published and widely reproduced, actual change is always different. Projections are only as good as their assumptions about fertility, mortality and

(sometimes) migration, and therefore of our understanding of recent trends. The perennial difficulty of population forecasters has been to anticipate fertility – in this century birth rates have been fickle. In comparison, demographers have in general seen mortality in steady decline, with the result that the accelerating decline of death rates in later life has been consistently underestimated. To add to this difficulty, the last decade has produced increases in British male death rates among young adults:

> For men between the ages of 24 and 46 mortality rates are tending to rise at present, largely due to deaths arising from HIV infection, but also from an increasing number of suicides and accidental deaths. ... Past and current trends suggest that those now over about age 47 will continue to show, in each cohort, lower mortality rates than in the preceding cohort ... this has been their experience to date and at present their mortality rates are diminishing by between one and four per cent a year.
>
> OPCS (1993) p. 8

Thus, a new difficulty faces forecasters, to anticipate the duration, pace and age distribution of mortality declines in old age, and to decide at what age the alteration to less favourable trends occurs. The 1991-based projections to 2031 (with extrapolations to 2061) use substantially revised assumptions for fertility: the assumed long-term family size for the UK has been reduced

Table 2.3: Age-specific death rates in England and Wales, 1901–92

Years	All ages	Age group (years)				
		0–1	55–64	65–74	75–84	85+
1901–05	16.0	138	28.7	59.4	127.3	258.6
1931–35	12.0	62	20.1	49.0	119.3	255.7
1961–65	11.8	21	15.8	39.6	96.7	220.2
1971–75	11.8	17	14.9	36.9	87.8	201.0
1981–85	11.7	10	13.4	33.4	78.2	186.3
1992	10.9	6.5	10.6	28.6	69.2	159.7
Annual rate of improvement (%)						
1843–93	0.3	–0.0	–0.3	–0.2	–0.1	0.2
1893–1953	0.8	2.8	1.1	0.8	0.5	0.3
1953–92	0.2	3.6	1.1	1.0	1.1	1.0
1983–92	0.8	4.7	2.6	1.7	2.6	1.7

Sources: OPCS (1989) *Mortality Statistics 1841–1985, Serial Tables.* HMSO, London, Table 1.
OPCS (1992) *Mortality Statistics 1990: England and Wales, General.* HMSO, London, Table 2.
OPCS (1994) *Mortality Statistics 1992: England and Wales, General.* HMSO, London, Tables 1 and 3.

Table 2.4: Projected number of elderly people by age in UK, 2001–61

Year	Population (× 1000)				Share of total (%)			Annual growth (%)*		
	60+	70+	80+	All ages	60+	70+	80+	60+	70+	80+
2001	12 204	6782	2520	59 719	20.4	11.4	4.2	0.2	0.8	1.6
2011	13 937	7135	2854	61 110	22.8	11.7	4.7	1.3	0.5	1.3
2021	15 764	8726	3200	61 980	25.4	14.1	5.2	1.2	2.0	1.2
2031	18 097	10 011	4288	62 096	29.1	16.1	6.9	1.4	1.4	3.0
2041	17 879	11 365	4817	60 987	29.3	18.6	7.9	−0.1	1.3	1.2
2051	17 450	10 647	5375	59 273	29.4	18.0	9.1	−0.2	−0.7	1.1
2061	17 105	10 251	4731	57 418	29.8	17.9	8.2	−0.2	−0.4	−1.3

*Average annual growth rate over previous decade.
Source: OPCS (1993) *National Population Projections 1991-based*. HMSO, London, Appendix I.

from 2.00 to 1.90 children per woman. A selection of the official projections is given in Table 2.4. They demonstrate the effects on the nation's age structure of:

- the present low level of fertility continuing

- the 'wave' effect of the high 1950s and 1960s birth cohorts being followed by the low birth cohorts of the 1970s and 1980s

- the increased survival of people into their 80s and 90s.

The 1990s will see a lower growth rate of the older population than in any previous decade of this century (compare Tables 2.1 and 2.4). Beginning in the first decade of the next century, however, a period of higher growth rates begins. It does not manifest for the 70+ years population until the second decade, or for the 80+ years until the 2020s. The UK population aged 60+ years will exceed 12 million during the 1990s and in the early decades of the next century will enter a period of faster growth, to 15.8 million by 2021. During the 2030s the growth phase will end. It is expected that by 2061 the 60+ years population will have fallen to 17.1 million, by 6% from 2041. As a result of the low fertility assumption, during this period the total population is likely to be falling and the elderly population will continue to grow as a share of the total. In 2031 it is likely to form 29.1% of the total, and by 2061 to be 29.8%.

Although the presented numbers and percentages are impressively large, the rates of growth of the older population during the next half century will be considerably lower than during the middle decades of the present century. It is surprising to see that during the 2020s, the peak

decade for the 'surge' of the 80+ years population, the annual rate of increase is likely to be lower than for the same age group during the 1930s and 1940s. An increasing average age is projected among the elderly population, and the numbers aged over 75 years and over 85 years are likely to grow more quickly than the entire elderly population.

Morbidity in later life

Average life expectancy has increased substantially during this century in developed countries but there is no firm evidence that the maximum possible lifespan has increased. A French lady recently died at 122 years of age, so the textbook maximum of 117 years must be revised, but the new record can be ascribed to probability and does not demonstrate that human physiology has changed. A majority of the population in affluent nations is now expected to achieve nearly 80 years, i.e. two-thirds of the maximum possible. Nearly 100% survive childhood and early adult decades. In great contrast to a century ago, the survival curve only begins to fall markedly after 50 years of age, but then it falls precipitately. Deaths have been concentrated into old age. In the UK in 1990, of the 327 198 female deaths, nearly a third (101 421) were of women aged 85 years or more, and 85% occurred at ages of 65 years or more.

The vital questions are whether the prevalence of sickness and functional restrictions is also being delayed and whether their duration has changed. Are successive cohorts healthier, with a later onset of disabling and lethal conditions? Or does a combination of greater vigour and more effective medical care prolong the duration of sickness and functional restriction? The debate about whether or not a 'compression of morbidity' is occurring has been vigorously pursued for more than a decade. Unfortunately, no country has adequate morbidity data over a sufficient time to provide an incontestable answer to these questions. The latest British evidence gives conflicting answers. If we rely on people's self-report of a limiting long-term illness (as asked in the national census and the *General Household Survey*), then it appears that unhealthy years have increased more than healthy years. If, however, data on more specific disabilities are analysed, the opposite conclusion is reached. Whichever is correct, the more substantial influence in the short term is likely to be the health service expectations of the population. All age groups are consulting their general practitioners more often and making increasing demands upon the acute services. This may have as much to do with a spreading awareness of the capabilities of modern medicine than with the intrinsic health of the population.

Regional variations

One final aspect of population trends should be more widely appreciated in health service management and by clinicians. The population is continuously redistributing within the country.

For most of the last half-century, the dominant trend was decentralization from larger cities. Older people participate in these shifts no less than other age groups, through their past decisions of where to live and work, and through migrations in later life.

The changes are shown by the projected rates of increase of two age groups of elderly people during 1993–2001 (Table 2.5). The variations in the 60–74 years population are not large: all regions are forecast to experience losses of 2.5 to 4.7%. Greater variation is anticipated in the forecasted change of the 75+ years population, but in all Regions at least 8% growth is forecast. When, however, the large metropolitan areas are separated (the righthand column in Table 2.5), then larger differences are expected. For the young elderly population, the range is from 'no change' in the extra-metropolitan areas of the Northern and Yorkshire & Humberside Regions to a 9% loss in Inner London and Tyne and Wear (i.e. Newcastle, Gateshead and Sunderland). For the older elderly population, the range is from a small loss in Inner London to a one-fifth increase in the northern extra-metropolitan areas. Population changes will not therefore impact on all regions and districts equally. For the foreseeable future, several metropolitan areas can expect continuing decreases in their elderly populations, and it is only in certain 'growth areas' around,

Table 2.5: Projected change in two age groups of older people in England, 1993–2001

Region	Change (%)		Sub-division	Change (%)	
	60–74	75+		60–74	75+
North	–3.4	18.4	Tyne and Wear MC	–9.1	15.0
			Remainder of the Region	0.0	20.4
North West	–4.7	9.1	Greater Manchester MC	–6.6	6.6
			Merseyside MC	–6.2	7.3
			Remainder of the Region	–1.8	12.6
Yorkshire & Humberside	–3.3	13.2	South Yorkshire MC	–6.3	12.8
			West Yorkshire MC	–4.5	10.1
			Remainder of the Region	0.0	20.4
East Midlands	–4.0	15.9			
West Midlands	–4.6	14.7	West Midlands MC	–8.5	11.9
			Remainder of the Region	–0.7	17.4
East Anglia	–2.5	18.9			
South East	–3.2	8.0	Greater London County	–7.9	–0.1
			Inner London	–8.9	–0.5
			Outer London	–7.4	0.1
			Remainder of the Region	–0.6	12.5
South West	–4.2	16.9			

but removed from, the large cities that rates of increase will be very high.

Conclusion

Contrary to many popular accounts, the rate of change of Britain's age structure towards an older population has slowed from its highest rates during the middle decades of the century. There will be another 'surge' that peaks during the third decade of the next century, as the high birth cohort of the 1960s reaches the retirement years, but the anticipated rates of growth in the 2020s will not match those we have already accommodated. And after 2030 (as few alarmist commentaries admit), the elderly population is likely to decrease for at least three decades.

For more than a century, the British population has benefited from progressive improvements in survival, although not in every age group in every decade. The annual decrease in infant deaths has been by far the fastest improvement, and is still rising, to more than 4.5% during each year of the 1980s. As in the US, a new feature of the last quarter century has been a marked decrease in mortality at the oldest ages. This brings about faster than recently projected rates of increase of the population in advanced old age. But the latest mortality trends are confounded by evidence of rising mortality among young men. This development has received relatively little comment in Britain to date, perhaps in the hope that it is a brief aberration. But if the worsening trend continues over another two decades, then much of the current alarm about the consequences of improving mortality at very great ages will appear capricious. The current climate of alarm and concern about ageing trends has little to do with demography, and is instead founded in rising health care and old age income demands, and in the political, ideological and professional responses they induce. Most professions welcome increasing demands for their services: it might be

instructive for clinicians and professional carers to see the health services' prospects in this light.

Key points

- The number of people surviving to old age is determined by birth, death and migration rates over more than six decades.

- Average period life expectancy at birth in 1991 in England and Wales was 79.0 years for women and 73.4 years for men.

- Nearly 16% of the population were aged over 65 years in 1996. Survival to old age has increased greatly in the 20th century, mainly as a result of decreased infant mortality.

- The numbers of older people in coming years will increase in some decades and fall in others, rather than rise relentlessly.

Further reading

Accessible recent accounts of population ageing include the following:

Central Health Monitoring Unit (1992) *The Health of Elderly People: An Epidemiological Overview, Volume 1* and *Companion Papers*, HMSO, London.

Grundy E (1992) The epidemiology of aging, in *Textbook of Geriatric Medicine* (eds Brocklehurst JC, Tallis RC, Traske K), 3rd edn. Churchill Livingstone, Edinburgh.

Olshansky SJ, Carnes BA and Cassel CK (1993) The aging of the human species. *Scientific American*, **268(April)**:18–24.

CHAPTER 3

The presentation and management of physical disease in older people

Sebastian Fairweather

Presentation

While in many instances disease in even very old people is little different than in those of middle age, the presentation of disease in older people can sometimes be obscure and its management complex. This chapter highlights some of the ways a different approach to older people may yield dividends by illustrating the presentation, diagnosis and management of some specific conditions. This is not a comprehensive account of medicine in old age, and certainly not a substitute for a standard general medical text to which the reader should refer when necessary.

Older people often delay in consulting a doctor because they associate their symptoms with ageing itself, or are reluctant to 'bother the doctor', or may not understand the benefits to be gained from modern treatments, or think doctors may be less willing to help older people. Nevertheless, there are organic reasons for failure to report symptoms, examples of which are listed in Box 3.1.

Box 3.1: Reasons for failure to report symptoms

- Poor memory or confusion (symptoms there but not reported)
- Normal memory but old person:
  - becomes used to symptoms, especially if long standing
  - regards symptoms as associated with ageing and thus incurable
  - recognizes significance, but frightened to seek medical help (typically worried about cancer or dementia)
  - fails to recognize significance of symptoms
- Physical adaptation or alteration in lifestyle to avoid provoking the symptoms (e.g. breathlessness)
- 'Genuine' lack of symptoms or signs (e.g. lack of fever, or appreciation of the cold, or altered pain perception)

Box 3.2: Major syndromes of non-specific presentation of physical illness in old age, 'IF OLD'

> **I**ncontinence
>
> **F**alls
>
> **O**ff **L**egs (immobility)
>
> **D**elirium (acute confusional state)

Older patients may also present in an apparently non-specific manner, which can be summarized by the acronym 'IF OLD' (see Box 3.2). Among the factors underlying such presentations are:

- the presence of multiple impairments often requiring rehabilitation

- multiple medical problems

- polypharmacy

- sensory, or cognitive, impairment leading to an inability to remember or recount an accurate history

- rapid deterioration if untreated

- complications of disease and therapy more common than in young and middle-aged patients.

One of the reasons for the non-specific presentation of disease is that the patients, and others, may express the problem in what seems to be social terms. For example, heart failure may present as needing help with shopping (for which a referral to a social worker rather than a doctor might seem appropriate) rather than breathlessness, or Parkinson's disease with incontinence as a result of poor mobility. Most standard medical texts emphasize impairment, whereas the elderly in the community emphasize disability and handicap.

An acute change in disability will almost certainly be due to a physical illness, although it may be difficult to uncover. This also emphasizes the importance of a simple objective way of measuring disability, for example the Barthel Index of activities of daily living (see page 116). Regular recording of this type of information, for example at an annual health check, will provide a useful baseline on which to assess changes, and importantly, give objective information on which to base realistic rehabilitation goals after illness.

Management

It is the doctor's aspiration to cure, but sometimes with elderly patients the main aim is avoiding deterioration, maintaining independence and relieving suffering. In every major medical contact there should be a process involving the following steps:

- undertake a comprehensive assessment, including

  - review of past problems
  - review of the social circumstances
  - meticulous physical examination
  - relevant investigations (see Box 3.3)

- formulate and agree a realistic goal and a management plan with all the appropriate parties. An assessment of pre-morbid independence is often helpful (hence the value of a routine Barthel score)

- implement the plan

- measure whether goals are being achieved (in the case of stroke rehabilitation, for example, regular use of Barthel score will show progress, and which items represent particular hurdles)

- review the plan, consulting and working with other members of the interdisciplinary team.

Factors underlying the ability to carry out this management plan include the following.

- How certain are you that disease is present?

- How severe is it?

- What stage or subtype of this disease are you dealing with?

- To what treatment is it likely to respond or what treatment should be given or will be accepted?

- What is the prognosis?

Box 3.3: Reasonable 'routine' investigation of illness in the home or surgery

- Relevant to infection:
  - accurate temperature recording (rectal 45 secs, or 10 mins under arm)
  - white blood cell (WBC) count: often a bit lower in older patients, normal result does not exclude infection
  - C-reactive protein (CRP): rises within 12–24 hours in bacterial infection
  - erythrocyte sedimentation rate (see text for discussion of ESR)
  - urinalysis for nitrite and WBCs
- Other tests:
  - haemoglobin and indices reduced in many major illnesses; primary screen for vitamin B_{12} and folate deficiency
  - albumin as a marker of illness
  - ECG (to exclude painless myocardial infarction)
  - serum: Na (if < 125 mM/l likely to be symptomatic); K (if < 3.0 mM/l likely to be symptomatic); urea (and creatinine) (measure of dehydration)*
    T4/TSH   hypothyroidism
  - Ca^{2+} – hypercalcaemia/cancer[†]
  - chest radiograph – heart size,[‡] heart failure, tumours, TB

* The urea/creatinine ratio is useful for assessing dehydration and over-diuresis in the old
† Mild asymptomatic hypercalcaemia is not uncommon in old women
‡ A CXR may be the most effective way to monitor the progress of CHF, particularly in the presence of obstructive airways disease

- How will you know that it is responding to treatment?
- How certain are you that other significant disorders have been excluded?

There is an understandable tendency to treat older patients less actively, whereas for the most part they need more attention to detail and more aggressive therapy than the young because their morbidity and mortality and response to many forms of treatment may be less marked. However, there may be circumstances where active intervention is not appropriate.

Management plan

A management plan should involve measures to:

- correct the primary defects
- maintain other functions (notably fluid and food)

- maintain a safe and appropriate environment (taking particular care to avoid falls)
- avoid preventable complications, such as pressure sores and venous thrombosis.

Unexplained illness

Lateral thinking may help when dealing with a curiously ill older person, or with something that does not quite 'fit'. Spontaneous hypothermia has been mentioned in this context. Also, think of some form of poisoning (in addition to the regular prescribed medication). Carbon monoxide poisoning is more common among those in low cost, poorly maintained housing; headaches, intermittent confusion and odd behaviour may be the only pointers. Very occasionally a leaky refrigerator may cause illness, as may any manner of household poisons. Remember also deliberate self-harm (which the individual will wish to hide) and harm from others, either in the form of outright abuse: physical (in the form of unexplained injuries); or chemical (in many forms including those beloved by crime writers). No social class, or personality type is immune from abuse. Indeed, on average, abuse is often perpetrated by a caring relative. Injuries for which the patient cannot give a convincing explanation, particularly around the face and upper arm, should raise suspicion; suspected abuse in an institution requires immediate and detailed investigation.

Anaemia

The need to mention the clinical diagnosis of anaemia was underlined for the author recently when one regular patient, in her 90s, with recurrent anaemia attended clinic, and even after looking specifically, I was very surprised to find the measured haemoglobin (Hb) to be as low as 5.5 gm/dl. Old people often have a degree of chronic conjunctivitis which may conceal even a well-established anaemia. On the other hand, pale conjunctivae are a feature of heart failure and any condition with a poor cardiac output. In addition to looking in the eyes, it is wise to look for circum-oral pallor and pallor of the palms of the hands.

Iron-deficiency anaemia

A common problem is how far to investigate iron deficiency in old age. A long history, poor diet and negative or only very weakly positive faecal occult blood (FOB) tests point away from bowel cancer as a cause. Likewise, if both upper gastrointestinal (GI) symptoms respond and positive FOB tests become negative with anti-ulcer medication, this points away from gastric cancer, especially if an NSAID or aspirin has been used in the recent past.

Nevertheless, symptoms and bleeding from gastric cancer can be temporarily reversed by a histamine H2 blocker. Not many very old people would accept a major gastrectomy even for cancer, so in this group, at least, an initial trial of therapy may be justified. However, the development of minimally invasive laser surgery may change all this.

Occult bleeding is commonly due to angiodysplasia in the large bowel, but lesions can be present throughout the GI tract. There is said to be an association between angiodysplasia and aortic stenosis, and some improvement with oestrogens can occur in problematic cases. Older ladies sometimes hide bleeding per vaginam, or haematuria, though both have to be very substantial to cause iron deficiency. It is thought that iron absorption may be lower in older people and reduced acid secretion in the stomach has also been implicated.

Immunosuppression

In the UK severe immunosuppression is uncommon. However, multiple myeloma, with depression of normal immunoglobulins, and malnutrition (see below) would be the likeliest causes, after the normal iatrogenic one – corticosteroid use. Immune suppression should be considered with any unusual infection, and perhaps especially with a crop of herpes simplex or herpes zoster.

Key points

- Skin colour is often misleading in the diagnosis of anaemia – do a blood count

- Consider regular FOB testing and (?)sigmoidoscopy in all elderly people presenting with iron-deficiency anaemia

- After an unusual, or viral, infection consider conditions causing immuno-suppression

Heart disease

Hypertension

In the western world, both systolic and diastolic blood pressure (BP) tend to rise with age until about 65. The pattern is complex but does not rise with age at all in developing countries.[1] The reasons for the western age-associated rise in BP and essential hypertension (which may not be the same thing) are not clear but probably are associated with progressive changes in vascular compliance from the teenage years onwards. It is

Box 3.4: Some types of hypertension in old age

- **Labile** a marker for substantial cardiovascular risk; it is not known whether therapy is as beneficial as in essential hypertension
- **Systolic** carries substantial risk of stroke and cardiac failure which benefit from treatment[4]
- **Essential** sBP > 160 mmHg, dBP > 90 mmHg
- **Renal** renovascular disease becomes progressively more common in old age
- **Exogenous corticosteroids** this combines with renal changes in old age
- **Alcoholic**
- **Iatrogenic** e.g. sodium-retaining drugs e.g. NSAIDs
- **Antidepressants** a paradoxical effect of tricyclics and MAOi in some patients
- **Hypervitaminosis-D and milk alkali syndrome** (may become more important with widespread vitamin-D and calcium supplementation)

not sufficiently emphasized how important treating systolic hypertension is in preventing heart failure.[2] There is considerable interest in the Honolulu long-term follow-up data which show a strong relationship between mid-life systolic BP and later life impaired cognitive function,[3] but preliminary data from a Swedish study suggest that lowering BP in some elderly people may impair cognitive function.

Lowering BP rapidly in older people is seldom necessary and is potentially dangerous. Accelerated and very severe hypertension and even hypertensive crises do occur in the old and lowering BP gently over a period of days is wise. Old people have a more variable BP than younger subjects and may be very hypertensive at some times and seriously hypotensive at others (see also the section on syncope and hypotension). There is reasonable concern that over-zealous lowering of BP may lead to nocturnal retinal ischaemia and accelerated loss of sight in those with glaucoma. Orthostatic hypotension is common in elderly hypertensives and exacerbated by most, if not all, drugs that lower BP.

Box 3.4 lists examples of the types of hypertension in older people. In some cases treatment will be of the underlying condition. Greater skill with renal angioplasty and the ready availability of the captopril renogram as a sensitive screening tool may make this form of treatment more important for the elderly in the future; it is certainly important to monitor renal function during therapy.

Guidelines for therapy

There is no proven benefit of treating hypertension in patients over the age of 85 years. It has become common practice to regard a BP of > 160/90 mmHg as hypertension for which treatment should be considered, and a BP of > 220/105 mmHg as severe hypertension normally requiring treatment. In a changing field perhaps it would be better to list circumstances which might alter the threshold for giving or withholding antihypertensives. These are given in Box 3.5. Conditions in the upper panel would give more cause for concern about the BP than in a person without these conditions; while with the conditions in the lower panel, BP would have to be very high before therapy was instituted.

Key points

- Treatment of hypertension in those over 85 years is still debatable
- Low-dose thiazide therapy is often effective on its own
- Use modest doses of drugs
- Orthostatic hypotension is commoner in hypertensives
- A 5 mmHg lowering of systolic BP confers a reduction in risk of stroke

Box 3.5: Guidance for blood pressure treatment

Conditions prompting need for tight control

Congestive heart failure

- **Renal impairment** – especially if progressive, but first check for severe renal artery stenosis

- **Diabetic** – control of other risk factors is particularly important in diabetics

- **Anticoagulants** – cerebral and other haemorrhage is more common with hypertension

- **Aortic aneurysm** – lowering BP will influence the rate of expansion. In this circumstance, drugs that lower aortic pressure most should be used notably ACEi and vasodilators (rather than diuretic and beta-blockers)

- **Ruptured cerebral berry aneurysm** – risk of rebleeding is partly related to systolic BP. Patients have a very high adrenergic drive, and beta-blockers may be particularly applicable

- **Intra-cerebral haemorrhage** – similar consideration as for ruptured aneurysm

- **Eye** – any operation in which the eye will be opened; hypertension carries an increased risk of catastrophic haemorrhage

Conditions demanding caution in lowering BP

- **Recent cerebral infarction** – most stroke patients will have a high BP which may settle by itself

- **Symptomatic orthostatic hypotension** – nearly all treatment will make it worse

- **Severe or poorly controlled glaucoma** – for fear of losing sight

- **Mental confusion** – lowering BP may worsen condition

Myocardial infarction

About half of all western men in their eighth decade have significant coronary artery disease. Older people generally suffer less pain with coronary thrombosis than younger people but truly silent myocardial infarction is less common than is generally believed among the old, where significant (even if temporary) impairment of myocardial function is likely to produce symptoms causing the patient to be listless, unable or unwilling to rise from bed or look after himself, or there may be arrhythmias or cardiac failure. Consequently, there is a case for an ECG in any non-specifically unwell older subject to rule out a major infarction.

Therapeutically this is important. Even if it is too late to consider thrombolysis, a large anterior infarct would prompt consideration of the use of anticoagulants to prevent or treat mural thrombosis to prevent systemic embolization. It should

at least suggest that an ECHO-cardiograph should be performed:

- to see if left ventricular thrombosis is present or

- to see if there is a substantial risk of future left ventricular thrombosis or

- to assess whether there is significant impairment of left ventricular systolic function such that the patient would benefit from ACE-inhibition or

- conversely whether he would be likely to tolerate a beta-blocker given prophylactically.

The use of aspirin is now widespread and in the domiciliary setting oral anti-coagulation with warfarin can be feasible, as may be the parenteral use of the newer heparin fragments which can be given twice daily subcutaneously with little or no monitoring. After myocardial infarction many older patients will require the use of an ACE-inhibitor (angiotensin converting enzyme inhibitor, ACEi) or perhaps the newer class of angiotensin-receptor blockers because of impaired systolic function. Secondary prevention may be just as relevant for the younger old as for middle-aged patients.

The benefits likely to be obtained from thrombolysis and more active treatment of myocardial infarction in old age are likely to be greater given the high mortality in old age, especially from an anterior infarct.

Cardiac rehabilitation

Many older patients will have some difficulty in looking after themselves in the immediate weeks after myocardial infarction as they adjust to impaired cardiac function and as left ventricular function recovers. It is probable that those living on their own, or who have to make significant physical effort in their own day-to-day care, have a higher mortality after myocardial infarction. It is important to assess the need for care, and to provide extra support for at least the first few weeks.

Older people may well benefit from the conditioning effect of controlled exercise, and this is also true of those with stable congestive heart failure (CHF). A substantial proportion of symptoms apparently related to cardiac dysfunction are in fact due to rapid and serious deconditioning of skeletal muscle. Indeed in severe cases this appears as a form of 'cardiac myopathy'. Graduated exercises may substantially improve this as well as giving confidence for a gradual return to a more normal life. Formal treadmill exercise testing may be helpful in showing when it is safe to proceed with more intensive exercise, although when used to screen elderly patients for reperfusion therapy it is less sensitive and less specific than in younger patients.[5]

Key points

- Painless myocardial infarction is common
- Old people have a greater benefit from thrombolysis than the young
- Ensure adequate support and rehabilitation after myocardial infarction

Congestive heart failure

Many older people adapt to, or become used to, chronic symptoms so that a classic story of orthopnoea or paroxysms of nocturnal dyspnoea may not be forthcoming; the patient may instead report insomnia. Effort dyspnoea is probably due to pulmonary congestion altering the mechanical work of breathing and it is most prominent in patients with difficulty in filling the left ventricle, those with pre-existing pulmonary disease or those with marked tachycardia or dysrhythmia with exercise. In patients with right ventricular failure, the lungs are to some extent protected from congestion. In these circumstances lethargy and exhaustion are more likely to be reported, or will be more dominant than dyspnoea.

The common causes of breathlessness, all of which are treatable, are:

- anaemia
- heart failure
- airways obstruction
- pulmonary embolization.

Less common causes include pulmonary fibrosis and infiltration of the lung by cancer.

Clinical diagnosis of heart failure

There are key features on examination which should be stressed.

- Is the heart enlarged?
  - a chest radiograph, or an ECHO-cardiograph may be necessary to assess this accurately
  - if the heart is not clearly enlarged do not be enthusiastic about diagnosing failure
- Is the jugular venous pulse (JVP) elevated?
  - this may be difficult to elicit, but if it is clearly elevated then right ventricular dysfunction is likely; most commonly secondary to chronic left ventricular dysfunction, but may be due to right ventricular ischaemia
- Is there peripheral oedema?
  - and if so, is there sacral oedema? Check for 'bilateral' pleural effusions

- Is there a prominent 3rd sound?
  - which suggests systolic dysfunction
- Is there a prominent 4th sound?
  - which suggests a stiff heart and diastolic dysfunction.

If two or more of the above features are present, then a diagnosis of heart failure is very likely. There is a strong argument for obtaining an ECHO-cardiograph on all new cases of heart failure and also in patients who have substantially deteriorated.

The probability of heart disease is more likely if the following are present:

- a long history of hypertension or ischaemic heart disease
- aortic and/or mitral valve disease
- a tachycardia.

An ECHO-cardiograph will help to establish the significance of myocardial function.

Management of congestive heart failure

The main management areas are listed.

- Improve systolic function.
- Reduce fluid overload.
- Consider dysrhythmias.
- Consider possibility of thrombo-embolic disease.
- Consider possibility of diastolic dysfunction.
- Give advice about nocturnal paroxysms.
- Consider long-term measures to improve function.

Improve systolic function

An ACE inhibitor (ACEi) should be tried such as captopril (starting with 6.25 mg) or the locally approved agent. If starting an ACEi after a diuretic the patient will need close supervision. A protocol needs to be agreed in practice in which ACE inhibition with a test dose of 6.25 mg captopril is preceded by a baseline BP measurement, the BP being monitored for an hour thereafter. Digoxin has a modest beneficial effect on systolic function and probably helps best the patients with severe dysfunction (tachycardia and prominent 3rd sound).

Reduce fluid overload

Diuretics remove excess sodium and water; begin with frusemide 20 or 40 mg daily. Bumetanide is better absorbed than frusemide and sometimes this is important. Long-term potassium supplements are only needed by the minority. Check serum potassium before initiation of treatment, then approximately weekly until stable. Do not routinely use a potassium-sparing agent in the old. If the patient resents a brisk diuresis (most prefer this to sphincter uncertainty in the day), switch to the thiazide combination, e.g. Dyazide or give a diuretic dose of say bendrofluazide 5 mg/day together with a routine potassium supplement because thiazides have twice the potassium depleting effect of loop agents. If digoxin is being used, monitor the potassium especially carefully as toxicity is greater in the presence of hypokalaemia.

Try to estimate a reasonable normal 'dry' weight for your patient and diurese down to achieve about this value. Check concurrent urea and creatinine, a rising urea creatinine ratio suggests dehydration. If in doubt clinically about how far to diurese, a repeat chest X-ray (CXR) will help assess pulmonary congestion. When airflow obstruction and congestive heart failure are both present, diurese the patient to normal lung fields on the CXR, and then tackle the airways with more intensive therapy if necessary.

Consider dysrhythmias

Atrial fibrillation should be controlled, or if of recent onset chemical cardioversion should be attempted. The possibility of paroxysmal arrhythmias should be considered. Digoxin partly controls atrial fibrillation by a central action mediated by the vagus nerve. In many old people digoxin may be less effective or ineffective in controlling the ventricular rate on exercise, and a second agent such as amiodarone may be needed, but its potentially serious side-effects cannot be ignored.

Consider possibility of thromboembolic disease

Give warfarin or aspirin for atrial fibrillation and remember that congestive heart failure patients are more prone to thrombo-embolic disease.

Consider possibility of diastolic dysfunction

If the ECHO-cardiograph shows good or reasonable systolic function your patient may benefit from a low dose beta-blocker (see below) or verapamil, but *not both* together.

Give advice about nocturnal paroxysms

A GTN spray and an extra-loop diuretic at night can help nocturnal spasms. These can be difficult to distinguish from nocturnal asthma.

Consider long-term measures to improve function

Patients with stable congestive heart failure may get long-term improvement from low-dose beta blockade, especially if there is an ischaemic component. The ECHO-cardiograph will help assess how safe this is. Surgery for functionally important valve lesions should be considered. Again, an ECHO-cardiograph will help decide which patients should be referred.

Remember congestive heart failure is a syndrome, not a 'specific disease entity', so in all cases consider ordering:

- ECG
- chest X-ray
- haemoglobin count
- thyroid function tests
- ECHO-cardiograph
- blood urea count
- electrolyte measures.

Heavy (alcoholic) drinking impairs cardiac function ('holiday heart').

Stroke

Incidence and prevalence

Stroke is one of the most common fatal or severely disabling conditions. It is responsible for the death of about 2% of all persons over 85 years every year (or about 15% of all deaths in this age group) as opposed to the annual death of about 0.1% of the 65 to 75 age group. The incidence and prevalence of all strokes is much higher than this, with severe stroke occurring in 13 per 100 000 total population; so each general practitioner (GP) could expect to have three patients in need of permanent nursing care as a result of stroke and about twice that number in need of substantial on-going care at home.

Presentation

The presentation of stroke merits special consideration. Lesions outside the main motor and sensory systems may present diagnostic difficulties. Ataxia, paresis and anaesthesia are usually reported accurately, but dyspraxias and various agnosias and problems with spatial orientation may well be perplexing to patients, relatives and doctors alike. One problem area is the right parietal lobe which is commonly affected by carotid and middle cerebral artery territory lesions. In this circumstance, the patient may have a problem describing what is wrong, or may even flatly deny an obvious paresis. It is important to test the visual fields for visual inattention, using double-simultaneous stimulation, as well as testing for cutaneous inattention, for vertical extinction and for spatial orientation. In the latter case, asking the patient to draw a clock face has much to commend it as a quick test of a variety of cognitive functions.

It can be useful to record routinely some basic neurological tests, such as mental status, Activities of Daily Living (ADL) scores and weight to provide a reference against which to measure future change. The plantar responses are commonly extensor in older patients, so the finding of an abnormal response does not necessarily provide much useful information in the diagnosis of a suspected recent cerebral infarction unless the plantars were known to be flexor before.

Investigation

In the UK, only about half of strokes are currently admitted to hospital. With greater emphasis on community care and community rehabilitation, deciding who needs further assessment or investigation is not straightforward. The following are important considerations.

- Is there any reason to doubt the diagnosis?

- Is there evidence of a source of emboli?

- Should the patient have a brain scan to detect haemorrhage or carotid scan to detect surgically correctable carotid artery stenosis? (Current evidence would not support endarterectomy in patients over the age of 85 years.)

- Is there evidence of systemic disease to which the stroke might be secondary?

All patients should have an ECG, and have blood glucose, haemoglobin, ESR and CRP measured.

Management

General management principles include the following.

- Ensuring that the diagnosis is correct.

- Optimizing treatment of associated conditions, such as hypoxia, heart failure and diabetes mellitus.

- Assessing ability to drink and eat, and providing appropriate support.

- Performing a functional assessment and maintaining a safe environment.

- Preventing complications, such as deep venous thrombosis (paralysed legs should be supported with graduated pressure stockings and prophylactic anticoagulation should be considered), and treating intercurrent infection.

- Setting up an early rehabilitation programme.

Prevention of stroke

This is a very complex and important area. Box 3.6 lists some representative risk factors for stroke in order of importance. It has been estimated that reducing systolic BP by just 5 mmHg would cut the stroke rate by between 15 and 22%; anticoagulation for non-rheumatic atrial fibrillation reduce it by 10%; and optimal surgical therapy for carotid stenosis reduce it by 1%.[6] The risk of a second stroke in the elderly is about 10% in the first year, and about 5% per annum thereafter. There is therefore a major incentive to attend to secondary prophylaxis.

Box 3.6: Some risk factors for stroke

Factor	Relative risk
BP > 160/90	7
Previous transient ischaemic attack	5
'Binge' drinking	5
Congestive heart failure	5
Ischaemic heart disease	3
Physical inactivity	2.5
Diabetes mellitus	2.2
Smoking	2
Obesity	1.5

Dizziness

Dizziness is one of the most difficult symptoms to assess and manage in old age. Some degree of postural instability is an inevitable part of growing older.[7] Many patients use the term dizziness, or giddiness, to describe any sense of instability, and may assume that if they have fallen, they must have been giddy or dizzy, or both. It is very important to try to get the patient to distinguish dizziness from a sense of rotation, since this helps diagnosis.

Giddiness on lying down in bed (i.e. on putting the head back on the pillow) or in first sitting up strongly point to ageing changes in the vestibular system. These symptoms may be confirmed using Hallpike's manoeuvre. Some patients only exhibit nystagmus when their head is held in a specific position (usually lying flat, or with the neck extended, and the neck rotated in one direction). Many older people feel very giddy when bending forward (for example when looking into a low cupboard or oven). Giddiness on standing up suggests postural hypertension.

Management

Management is supportive and, where appropriate, treatment of the underlying condition. Reassurance may be all that is needed, and advising a stick or frame. Labarynthine sedatives sometimes help slightly, but can often make things worse. Avoiding abrupt movements, particularly movements of the head and neck can be most effective, and sometimes a soft cervical collar is helpful purely as a means of limiting movement.

Delirium

Confusional states are very important and quite common in elderly people. Indeed, almost any disease or disorder in older people can present as delirium. It can be an adverse marker normally associated with serious underlying disease. This subject is dealt with at length in Chapter 4.

Vision

Cataract, glaucoma, macular degeneration and diabetic retinopathy are all common in elderly people. Old-age reduction in pupillary size reduces the amount of light reaching the retina, and has an important effect on acuity. The prevalence of blindness is about 2% in the over 75s, and 0.4% in the 65–75 age group; the rates in people below this age are about ten times lower. The comparison rates for deafness are 30% for 65–75, and 50% above this age. Combined impairment of vision and hearing is therefore distressingly common among the very old.

Occasionally visual problems can present as a true or apparent confusional state. The basis of this is either the confusional effect of cortical blindness (or a visual agnosia) so that the subject is unaware that they are not seeing properly, or as a result of a painful eye condition. Acute glaucoma normally presents as an acute painful eye, but in patients with cognitive impairment any painful condition may not be accurately reported and may present as worsening confusion. Part of the normal examination of the older adult should include a simple test of visual acuity (such as reading a newspaper), assessment of the visual fields to confrontation and fundoscopy to assess the area of the optic cup (as a screening test for glaucoma). About 10% of newly diagnosed elderly diabetics will have detectable retinopathy.

While severe hearing impairment is hardly to be missed, it is necessary to test each ear individually because some patients can compensate with the 'normal' side remarkably well. The drums should also be inspected in a case of infection where the site is not certain; wax is a problem which is easy to deal with when the hearing is impaired.

The feet

The feet are often a rather neglected part of the overall assessment and examination of a patient. Ill-fitting shoes and painful feet are an important cause of locomotor difficulty in the old. Among women in particular, footwear is sometimes inappropriately light for someone with deteriorating balance. Bunions are common, and old people often have difficulty cutting ever-hardening nails. Neuropathy is common, as are claw toes, and alteration in the foot arches which can be uncomfortable and cause instability. Peripheral circulation is also often poor. Foot care is important for all but it is particularly important in diabetics who may easily develop penetrating ulcers.

The gastrointestinal tract

Mouth

A sore or infected mouth or ill-fitting or absent dentures will deter adequate fluid and food intake. Do not overlook inspection of the mouth – it is all too easily done.

Oesophagus

Some degree of difficulty in swallowing is quite common in very old people. Components in this may be failure to chew food adequately, reduced production of saliva (xerostomia), and poorly coordinated oesophageal contractions. Radio-labelled tagging has shown that accumulation of tablets in the low oesophagus is very common and therefore they should be taken in the upright position with an adequate bolus of fluid.

Stomach

Aside from the high age-associated incidence of gastric cancer, painless gastric ulceration is notable in old people. Giant gastric ulcers may cause weight loss in the absence of any other specific features. There is often an associated use of NSAIDs which may be the cause of ulcers in the jejunum, caecum and even colon, none of these will be seen on routine endoscopy or barium studies.

Malabsorption

Gluten enteropathy (coeliac disease) is being increasingly recognized in even the very old. Small bowel bacterial overgrowth sufficient to cause malabsorbtion appears to be quite common in old age, and occasionally giardiasis can be very difficult to diagnose without a small-bowel biopsy. The dilemma is how far to go in proving malabsorption and its cause. Careful weighing and monitoring a proven deficiency (e.g. folate) with a therapeutic trial of a broad-spectrum antibiotic (e.g. doxycycline and met-ronidazole) for four weeks is often justified because it will cure giardiasis and overgrowth, with the subsequent course suggesting whether a relapse in bacterial overgrowth is occurring. The 14C-xylose breath test is probably the easiest and most sensitive for diagnosing overgrowth but can be cumbersome for a frail subject living a long way from an investigation centre, which is why a sensibly managed therapeutic trial may be useful.

Nutritional deficiencies

A degree of weight loss is normal in old age; in the over 80s expect about 0.3% loss of body weight per year before considering it to be patho-logical. Lean body mass declines markedly but a rise in fat content may partially hide this. The crucial factor however, is noting a recent change. It is perfectly possible for the apparently obese to have dietary nutritional deficiencies while a subject with almost no subcutaneous fat may be replete in all essential nutritional elements. In those suspected of being undernourished an assessment should be made of:

- the patient's ability to obtain and prepare food

- cognitive function (weight loss is a feature of dementing illnesses) – check also for depression

- the oral cavity and ability to chew

- special search for factors in the oesophagus and upper GI tract which may impair food intake or absorption.

Osteomalacia

Among the nutritional deficiencies it is worth noting the non-specific presentation of osteo-malacia. Although overt osteomalacia has become uncommon in the western world, lesser forms of vitamin-D deficiency have been shown by surveys to be almost the rule in the housebound old. Proximal myopathy and a waddling gait may not be obvious and the patient may just complain of malaise, bone pain, or simply be more dependent. The diagnosis rests on measuring the serum calcium together with the albumin and serum phosphate and alkaline phosphatase (consult your local laboratory for reference ranges, and for a factorial formula to help integrate these). Plasma vitamin-D levels are difficult to measure and are anyway nearly always low in the frail old. Radiological signs (pseudo-fractures) are usually late. Osteomalacia in older people is almost always related to the combination of a diet low in vitamin-D and seldom exposure to sunlight. Indeed, possibly any older person who is housebound and does not take fortified foods should be given physiological vitamin-D supplements.

Overt osteomalacia should be treated by an intramuscular injection of 150 000 IU of cholecalciferol while a search is being made for malabsorption. This should be adequate replenishment for six months, and during this time a decision can be made as to whether oral absorption will be adequate or whether six-monthly injections will be required. The biochemistry and bone lesions in osteomalacia may persist for many months.

Vitamin-C, folate and other deficiencies

Vitamin-C deficiency and scurvy are uncommon, but is often atypical in the old, with sheet haemorrhages in the legs. Gastrointestinal bleeding may cause hypochromic iron-deficient anaemia. Modest folate deficiency seems to be quite common in the UK, especially in those with senile dementia; perhaps elderly patients self-select a relatively low folate diet, or gastrointestinal absorption may be low. It is tempting to think that under- or mal-nutrition can underlie some of the multiple problems from which frail older people living on their own seem to suffer, including for example, repeated infections. A crude measure of the likely dietary provision is the amount spent on food for the residents in nursing homes per week.

Weight loss and calorie intake

Reduced intake of food underlies nearly all cases of weight loss. Occasionally, patients will claim to be eating well, in which case one suspects hyperthyroidism or diabetes mellitus with the spillage of substantial calories in the form of glucose in the urine.

Key points

- Confirm weight loss by regular weighing (a base weight at annual health review)
- Weight loss is often a marker of poor care, depression and dementia
- Consider administering vitamin-D and calcium supplements

Large bowel

Constipation underlies many unexplained abdominal pains, and is also a major cause of faecal incontinence. While increased transit times are a feature of the ageing gut; dehydration, immobility from illness, and drugs such as analgesics and anticholinergic agents can cause severe constipation. An enquiry about the frequency of bowel opening is not adequate as even in severe constipation this may be daily or more. Rectal and abdominal examination is mandatory. Where there is a possibility of colorectal cancer, testing for faecal occult bloods and flexible sigmoidoscopy should be considered.

Inflammatory proctitis is relatively common, and normally responds readily to local steroids so that diagnosis is important: a protosigmoidoscopy, with biopsy, showing proctitis with normal mucosa above is usually sufficient. Gut ischaemia is a cause of colitis and needs to be remembered.

Key points

- Check the teeth
- Advise the taking of tablets with water, and not when lying down
- Peptic ulceration may not be painful
- Bacterial overgrowth may cause malabsorption
- Localized proctitis may cause diarrhoea

Hypothermia

This is defined as a core temperature below 35 °C. The lower the temperature, the greater the morbidity. In the 1960s, 0.68% of UK hospital admissions were associated with hypothermia. A large community study in the 1970s found a spontaneous hypothermia rate of 10% of those living alone.[8] However, it is likely that the prevalence is variable and is dependent on the ambient temperature in the home.

Factors causing hypothermia include:

- The environment
  - ambient temperature
  - quality and state of repair of housing
  - availability and use of heating
    (note that these two are not the same, and that temperature may vary a lot in one house)
  - wearing appropriate clothes (in many cases there is a poor adaptive response to cold)

- Pathological causes
  - immobility and falls
    (even young subjects may become rapidly hypothermic when lying still in a cold environment)
  - drugs
    (vasodilators such as chlorpromazine may lower temperature; drug-induced falls may secondarily do the same)
  - concurrent diseases, such as diabetes mellitus
    (diabetics have a six-fold increased risk of hypothermia; hypoglycaemia, whatever its cause, impairs shivering even in fit subjects)
  - intercurrent illness
    (this is the main cause probably by affecting heat production and conservation)

- Socio-economic factors
  - living alone
  - excessive alcohol intake
  - impaired mobility

- Physiological changes
  - low body mass
    (poorly nourished individuals may have difficulty in raising heat production)
  - autonomic impairment
    (many hypothermic individuals have been shown on recovery to have persisting relevant autonomic defects).

Diagnosis

Hypothermia usually occurs in a context which makes the possibility obvious. However, even in an English summer, the indoor temperature may be cold enough for an immobile older subject to lose heat rapidly. To the practised hand placed on the chest for percussion, or on the abdomen, the cold 'dead' feel of the hypothermic torso is unmistakable. In addition, the respiration rate may be slow and pulses barely palpable. A myxoedematous face may bring the possibility to mind. A normal oral, axillary or tympanic membrane temperature effectively excludes core-hypothermia, but a low temperature at these sites does not prove it. It is for this reason that a low-reading rectal thermometer is recommended. An ECG may reveal sinus bradycardia with some degree of atrioventricular block, or slow atrial fibrillation. J-waves (positive deflections at the QRS-ST segment junction) are highly specific but much less sensitive than the rectal temperature recording.

Key points

- Spontaneous hypothermia is rare, most cases will be secondary to severe illness
- Exclude diabetes, hypothyroidism and infections
- Social and environmental assessment is vital
- Hypothermia impairs judgement and performance
- Check drug therapy

The genitourinary system

Renal function deteriorates significantly with age from the fourth decade. Approximately 1 ml/min of the glomerular filtration rate (GFR) is lost per year of life, and an approximation for the current GFR is 140 minus age. Muscle mass and hence serum creatinine values tend to decline with age so that the normal range for serum creatinine is not the same in the very old as in the young. An approximation for GFR is given by:

$$GFR = \frac{(140 - age) \times weight\ (kg)}{serum\ creatinine\ (\mu mol)}$$

This decline in renal function has important implications for a variety of diseases, and for the use of drugs which are mainly excreted by the kidneys, such as gentamicin or digoxin. Renal failure has few specific features until it is advanced.

Key points

- Renal function declines substantially with age

- Serum creatinine by itself is an inadequate assessment of renal function in the old

- Beware of renally excreted drugs

Recurrent urinary infection

Recurrent urinary infection is a major problem for some older people, particularly females. Causes include failure to treat the initial infection adequately, presence of bladder stones, failure to void completely, oestrogen deficiency, urethral trauma and prostate enlargement. Frail older people can quickly become seriously ill and then require admission to hospital. Such infections are commonly associated with incontinence of urine.

The definition of recurrent infection is arbitrary, but some patients get into trouble every few weeks. To prevent recurrence it is essential to treat the infection adequately initially. There are no good trial data, but clinical experience suggests that single-dose antibiotics and bacteriostatic agents are associated with high recurrence rates. Other simple steps include avoiding long periods without fluid, and teaching double-voiding to ensure as complete bladder emptying as is possible. In women, oestrogen deficiency may be a significant factor and infection rate is reduced by the use of topical or oral oestrogen replacement. With older patients, intermittent courses of unopposed oestrogen, in physiological doses, may be used.

Catheter infections and blockage

Most long-term catheters become infected and this frequently leads to renal parenchymal infection which is why there has been a move to intermittent catheterization in younger patients. Catheter blockage is normally associated with heavy colonization. The length of time a urinary catheter will survive between blockages can be increased by ensuring a urine flow of at least one and a half litres of urine per day, and by measures which reduce urinary bacterial counts, such as using a urinary antiseptic or regularly drinking cranberry juice.

The prostate

Prostatic symptoms are very common, perhaps universal, in old age. The presentation and management of benign prostatic hyperplasia (BPH) is well dealt with in standard medical and surgical texts. A few points are emphasized here.

- BPH and changes in the bladder make the old more susceptible to drug-induced retention, e.g. by tricyclics.

- While most patients are aware of prostatic obstruction, some patients get significant retention (and renal failure) with few symptoms; (thus always check for hydronephrosis in an elderly man with renal impairment).

- Drug management of BPH (alpha-blockers and testosterone suppression) may be very effective and appropriate in the frail elderly or those at high operative risk.

- The prostate can be the site of occult infection, leading to mental confusion. Bacteria from the prostate can spread to the bones of the lumbar spine, in a similar manner to prostate cancer. This emphasizes the importance of rectal examination.

Cancer of the prostate

While more than 50% of very elderly men have histological cancer of the prostate, it will only become clinically evident in less than one third. However, it is the second most common cause of death from cancer in males over 75. At present, there is no treatment which has been shown to improve survival in asymptomatic patients, which suggests that screening such patients for cancer would not be useful. Nevertheless, the position may change if more effective therapy, or better ways of classifying prostate cancer are developed. A rectal examination is part of the full assessment of an elderly male, and extensive prostate cancer can usually be diagnosed by digital examination.

In recent years the prostate specific antigen (PSA) assessment has replaced acid serum phosphate in the diagnosis of carcinoma of the prostate but it is a test which must be used judiciously. There is for example no case for using it as a screening instrument at present since nothing is gained by establishing the diagnosis earlier, no current treatment is available and using a PSA for screening purposes produces a worrying number of false positive results.

Any finding of over 4 ng/l *may* be abnormal especially if rectal examination raises suspicions of carcinoma of the prostate and the predictive value of the test in these circumstances would be between 15 and 20%. This figure rises to 80% when the PSA exceeds 20 ng/l. PSA measurements may also be useful in the diagnosis of extensive dissemination of prostatic cancer. This is, however, a changing field and local guidelines should be followed.

Key points

- Treat urinary infection, especially if recurrent, vigorously

- Think of oestrogen deficiency in women

- Prostatic cancer may present with backache

- Malaise in an old man may be due to chronic retention and renal failure

- Request and interpret the PSA with great care – it is not currently a screening instrument

---

The American Cancer Society recommends digital examination of the prostate per rectum every year in men aged over 40 years.

Immobility

The causes of immobility are often diverse in any one patient. Adequate assessment is therefore essential.

Assessment of a poorly mobile subject

- Is there a simple painful explanation?
  e.g. fracture, spondylosis, arthritis or myalgia, or problems with the feet.

- Is there a problem with neuromuscular function?
  For example, muscular weakness (e.g. myopathy, neuropathy, hemiplegia or paraplegia).

- Is there a problem with 'co-ordination'?
  e.g. a drug-induced defect, Parkinson's disease, cerebellar ataxia, gait dyspraxia such as with normal pressure hydrocephalus, or severe sensory disturbance.

- Is there a circulatory factor?
  e.g. severe effort dyspnoea, orthostatic or exertional hypotension, acute myocardial infarction.

- Is the immobility a manifestation of a severe constitutional illness? (of which infection would be the commonest).

- Are there psychological factors?
  For example, a fear of falling, or depression, or attention-seeking behaviour (although the latter would be very unusual unless part of a prolonged background of similar behaviour).

Being able to stand requires that the lower limb muscles generate enough force to counteract the force of gravity on body mass which may be excessive. An octogenarian may need to use 90% of his peak quadriceps muscle power to rise unaided from a chair. Just a short time in bed will rob him of sufficient strength to get up, as might a mild attack of arthritis in a knee. Likewise, a modest electrolyte disturbance may make the patient just weak enough to be immobile. As a rule, if a patient has enough strength to lift his legs off the bed (when lying down) he has enough strength to stand and walk, at least slowly.

A cerebellar syndrome of sufficient severity to prevent walking should be obvious, but bear in mind pure truncal ataxia. Extra-pyramidal defects and gait apraxias (due to frontal lesions) are often less obvious. Older people may have extra-pyramidal defects that are far from typical and may predominantly affect the axial muscles or lower limbs and therefore are less evident when the hands are examined.

Every patient should have their blood pressure measured lying and standing and at the point when they feel they can no longer walk. Exertional hypotension can be very severe and is commonly drug induced.

Management

Management is obviously that of the underlying condition(s). Mobility restriction has major implications for self-care, and the Barthel score may be a helpful means of assessing the need for extra help in the home, especially in more disabled subjects. Alterations to the home, the provision of commodes and walking aids may be necessary; and the advice of a community occupational therapist may be very helpful.

Key points

- Immobility is often multifactorial

- A detailed examination is necessary

- A thorough appraisal of the environment and involvement of an occupational therapist and a physiotherapist can be important

Incontinence

Up to 15% of young women will admit to inappropriate passage of some urine within the previous month.[9] Elderly people in the community may report a 30% involuntary urine loss rate, and in institutional dwellers, the rate may be over 50%. The male/female prevalence is about 1 : 2. There is no doubt that urinary problems and a fear of urinary problems are a major issue for many older people.

Box 3.7: Incontinence of urine

- Functional
  - cannot reach the lavatory in time (or at all)
  - in an unfamiliar environment
  - greater than normal urine flow (e.g. diabetes or diuretics)

- Failure to recognize need to void
  - delirium
  - drug intoxication
  - frontal lesion
  - normal pressure hydrocephalus
  - dementia

- Failure of control
  - overflow (continual dribbles)
  - severe detrusor instability (irregular large volumes, often in association with functional incontinence, but if acute consider urinary infection)

- Sphincter defects
  - mechanical (e.g. stress incontinence – small leaks in association with changes in intra-abdominal pressure – it is important to get the patient to strain during examination)
  - neuropathy (e.g. in lumbar stenosis, or with diabetes)

Causes (see Box 3.7)

There are centres concerned with bladder function in the frontal lobes, brain stem (pontine) and spinal cord (S2,3 and 4). Damage to higher centres generally leads to detrusor overactivity, resulting in the syndrome of urgency. The crucial factor here is the reduction in the time between the first sensation of the need to void and an irresistible detrusor contraction and uncontrolled voiding. This usually results in the passage of a bladder full of urine. Initially, this results in flooding incontinence, but as the condition worsens the functional bladder capacity is less and the volume voided is therefore smaller. This is usually prominent at night and severe urgency without nocturia or nocturnal incontinence should raise suspicion of a psychological disorder.

Damage to lower centres may give rise to the syndrome of detrusor-sphincter-dyssynergia where the external sphincter fails to relax properly with a voluntary voiding effort leading to inability to empty the bladder in the face of urgency. The subject may void on standing up or soon after making an ineffectual attempt to void seated. This may lead to accusations of wilfulness which will be distressing for the patient. Drugs which inhibit the external sphincter (such as alpha-adrenergic blockers) may be helpful, although they are prone to adverse effects and may exacerbate associated urge incontinence.

Damage in the spinal cord or in lower neurones (for example in diabetic neuropathy) may give rise to a low-pressure, hypotonic bladder without sensation. This will lead to overflow or dribbling incontinence. On examination the bladder should be palpable, although an ultrasound may be necessary to detect a non-tense, low-pressure bladder. Serious bladder outlet obstruction will also lead to dribbling although in this case, initially at least, the bladder should be tense, palpable or even tender, although with very long standing retention, an atonic bladder may develop.

Damage to the outflow sphincter may produce a type of dribbling incontinence. In women, descent of the bladder neck below the pelvic sling will produce stress incontinence; that is the passage of small quantities of urine with elevation in intra-abdominal pressure. This is usually very easy to distinguish from urge incontinence, although when very severe, urgency may appear like stress incontinence; the previous history should make matters clear.

Diagnosis and differential diagnosis

A simple practical approach to the problem of incontinence in old age is shown in Box 3.8, although in such a complex area this approach may be disputed. In any event, incontinence is often multifactorial. Box 3.9 lists some practical steps which should be undertaken in the surgery. Much controversy exists as to the role of invasive urodynamics in the diagnosis of incontinence. It is the author's opinion that the majority of cases can be diagnosed without recourse to anything but the simplest investigations. There are some clinical points which should be emphasized.

An understanding of the mechanisms of incontinence and an accurate history supplemented by an independent witness (because patients are often coy about the sphincters) and sometimes charting of the pattern of micturition are the key. Enquiries about possible neurological disturbances and a recent bowel history are mandatory, as is a neurological examination including testing perianal sensation and a digital rectal examination. Significant retention can be excluded by a one-off catheterization after a determined effort to empty the bladder. Although this is more invasive than ultrasound, it can be performed in the home and save a long journey and wait for a frail elder. Incontinence of urine is often an incidental part of serious illness which may include delirium and immobility, but this should be obvious. Incontinence is often unreported by the patient. This occasionally may be due to cognitive and memory impairment, but for many patients, losing control of the sphincters is so degrading and such a portend of impending senile decline as to be concealed. Fear of incontinence often leads older people to change their lifestyle radically, particularly with reference to going out, and also to reduce their fluid intake, sometimes to dangerous levels.

Management

Although management must depend upon the cause, as there is frequently more than one pertinent factor the approach will be multi-faceted. The following are some areas to cover.

- The environment
  - ensure that access to a toilet is easy. Often just providing a bedside commode is all that is necessary.

Box 3.8: Simplified algorithm for the differential diagnosis and management of urinary incontinence

Infection?   *yes* ——→   treat and review

no ↓

Diuresis?   *yes* ——→   modify drugs/treat diabetes

no ↓

Obstructed?   *yes* ——→   treat constipation, review drug chart, refer for advice

no ↓

Clear evidence of stress?   *yes* ——→   start stress-INCU programme

no ↓

Abdominal gait?   *yes* ——→   investigate for central lesions

and/or ↓

Abnormal perianal sensation?   *yes* ——→   Investigate for spinal lesion

no ↓

Clear evidence of urgency?   *yes* ——→   start urge-INCU programme

no ↓

Refer for advice

Box 3.9: Simple practical steps to be taken in a case of urinary incontinence

- Exclude UTI – dip-stick the urine. This is rarely the sole cause of incontinence but often contributes to an exacerbation

- Exclude heavy glycosuria – dip-stick the urine. This does not exclude diabetes mellitus in the old because of a rising renal threshold, nor does it exclude diabetic neuropathy; but it will exclude a sugar osmotic diuresis as a cause of incontinence

- Exclude retention (males) – a pelvic post-micturition ultrasound may be needed; a normal prostate on rectal examination does not rule out an obstructed bladder

- Exclude/treat constipation – rectal examination is mandatory; double incontinence is almost always due to faecal impaction

- Consider potential offending drugs – tricyclic antidepressants and opiates cause constipation

---

- Mobility
  - improve mobility as much as possible.

- Cognitive function
  - ensure the toilet is adequately signed and help is available.

- Drug list
  - keep diuretics to a minimum
  - review constipating, anti-cholinergic, anti-alpha-adrenergic, calcium-channel blocking drugs, or medication likely to cause confusion

– consider drugs which may help some aspects of bladder function (see below)
– check agents that may irritate the bladder.

The main incontinence syndromes may be managed as follows:

• if the main problem is overflow obtain specialist advice

• if the main problem is stress incontinence, consider: containment pads (they may work if the voided urine is less than 200 ml per episode); oestrogen replacement; pelvic floor exercises; surgical repair

• if the main problem is urge incontinence, consider: oestrogen replacement (in a female); in a robust subject, a type-A toileting regimen (see below); in a frail subject, a type-B toileting regimen (see below); bladder sedative drugs (see below) especially for nocturnal incontinence

• if the main problem is nocturnal incontinence, consider: that nocturnal polyuria may be the culprit; bladder sedative drugs (see below).

Drugs

A variety of drugs affects the function of the urinary bladder. These may have a direct effect on the detrusor muscle (e.g. flavoxate), or on the external sphincter as well (e.g. alpha-blocking drugs), or on the nerves supplying the lower urinary tract. Anti-cholinergic drugs can have a marked effect in reducing detrusor contraction, and might be expected to have a major role in the management of urge incontinence. Unfortunately, with urge incontinence the crucial thing is usually not the frequency of voiding but the duration of the warning of an impending void. Anti-cholinergics seem to shorten this period in many patients and so may make incontinence worse, quite apart from precipitating urinary retention. At night this is not a problem and anti-cholinergic drugs can be expected to reduce nocturnal frequency by increasing bladder capacity. The tricyclic antidepressants, especially Imipramine, also have an adrenergic-like effect in increasing the external sphincter tone and this is probably why they are the most effective agents in relieving urge incontinence

and in precipitating urinary retention in susceptible males. Imipramine 25–50 mg at night can be expected to reduce nocturnal frequency, but will not render a very frequent wetter completely dry.

Alpha-adrenergic blocking drugs, by contrast, reduce external sphincter tone and can relieve symptoms from bladder outflow obstruction. Consequently they will make urge incontinence worse. They can be useful for patients with detrusor-sphincter-dyssynergia and occasionally there may be merit in combining this with a pure anti-cholinergic (i.e. not Imipramine) in patients with mixed dyssynergia and instability. This should be done with specialist advice. They can also be useful in patients with marked prostatism.

Type-A toileting regimen

The object of this regimen is to retrain the bladder to accept larger volumes of urine. This is perhaps analogous to surgical bladder dilatation which can also be effective. In this regimen a pattern and frequency of regular voiding is chosen sufficient to keep the patient confident and dry. The patient is then required to increase gradually the times between the voids in very small steps, say by five minutes every week with an absolute prohibition on voiding before the predetermined time. Over a period of several months, an acceptable pattern may be achieved, but this requires great perseverance. The author does not recommend this approach for the frail elderly, or for those with significant neurological disease. It is probably best for those in whom the instability is either wholly or partially psychological.

Type-B toileting regimen

The object of this regimen is quite the opposite from the above: that is simply to keep the bladder volume below that which triggers a voiding contraction. Thus the patient is required to void on a regular basis just sufficiently often to prevent involuntary urination. The frequency and pattern will depend on the severity of the instability and the pattern of fluid intake but may need to be as often as every two hours by day. Strict adherence to an appropriate regimen will keep any patient with pure urgency dry providing they are able to empty the bladder.

Box 3.10: Incontinence of faeces

- **Functional** cannot reach the lavatory in time; often in an unfamiliar environment; greater than normal faecal volume; impaction with overflow; any cause of diarrhoea (NB laxative abuse)

- **Failure to recognize need to void**
  - delirium
  - drug intoxication
  - frontal lesion
  - dementia

- **Failure of control**

  - proctitis (this is not rare, proctoscopy is required)
  - sphincter defects (get the patient to strain, a prolapse may be intermittent)

Much can be done to help the incontinent patient and the pessimistic attitude of some doctors to this problem is quite unjustified.

Incontinence of faeces

Incontinence of faeces (see Box 3.10), in almost all cases, calls for one immediate investigation: a rectal examination. This examination will reveal the presence of:

- gross anatomical lesions (prolapse etc.)

- an impaired anal reflex (contraction of the anal ring on stroking the perianal skin)

- reduced anal tone (get the patient to squeeze your finger)

- impaction.

A full rectum in the context of incontinence, without an obvious diarrhoeal illness, should be treated as impaction in the first instance. If the rectum is empty, feel the descending and transverse colon. If the rectum is empty and the colon impalpable (in a not too-well covered individual) then a higher impaction (e.g. caused by an obstructing lesion such as a cancer or stricture) is unlikely. If you are uncertain after examination, a plain abdominal radiograph may help, but in domiciliary practice it may be easier to treat for impaction than send a patient for an X-ray. The continued faecal leakage typical of impaction may not be loose enough to be categorized as diarrhoea, but the stool, in these circumstances, is never formed. Indeed, incontinence of faeces with a normal formed stool strongly suggests a central neurological defect, usually in the frontal lobes.

Double incontinence is either the result of a gross neurological defect, which will be obvious, or faecal impaction sufficient to interfere with the external bladder sphincter – this will be obvious to the practitioner who carries out a rectal examination.

Management

Faecal impaction should be dealt with vigorously with laxatives and enemas; a severely impacted patient may take a week or more of daily enemas to clear out. Sphincter disturbances should be referred for specialist advice. Once the bowel has been cleared the patient should be given general advice on diet to prevent recurrence.

If treatment fails to establish faecal continence then soiling can be avoided by modest constipation and regular enemas to enable the bowels to be cleared out at a regular time. Codeine phosphate 30 mg once or twice daily with enemas two or three times per week are often successful. With this regimen, the bowels need to be monitored to avoid severe constipation from the drugs.

Key points

- A rectal examination is mandatory

- Faecal incontinence can almost always be controlled

- Faecal impaction should always be kept in mind

The musculoskeletal system

Osteoarthrosis

The commonest form of joint disease in old age is osteoarthrosis, which is an almost universal affliction of the over 50s.

Osteoarthrosis usually causes chronic pain and some joint stiffness on moving. Arthritis of the spine (spondylosis) may cause root pain through nerve entrapment. In addition, osteoarthrosis may have acute 'flare-ups', for no obvious reason, with inflammatory cells present in the synovial fluid. This usually responds to oral non-steroidals, or intra-articular corticosteroid. Chronic stable osteoarthrosis is better treated by simple analgesia.

Management of severe back pain in the old

Patients are occasionally crippled by the most debilitating back pain, either from degenerative changes or from osteoporotic vertebral collapse. Sometimes such patients have to be admitted to hospital but intensive management of pain at home should be possible. The elements of care are:

- to keep the patient in the most comfortable position and to avoid provoking pain

- paracetamol 1.0 g four times daily, regularly

- NSAIDs such as ibuprofen 400 mg, three times daily (or a stronger agent with cytoprotection)

- laxative (e.g. lactulose 20 ml twice daily, to prevent straining and constipation)

- imipramine 10 mg, twice daily as an analgesic adjuvant (amitriptyline is more sedating)

- codeine 30 mg, as necessary or if the pain is very severe or; morphine sulphate, starting with 2.5 mg orally, every four hours.

Management of osteoarthrosis

Management of joint pain includes:

- weight loss (especially for osteoarthritic knees)

- local creams (such as NSAIDs and capsaiah ointment)

- simple analgesia (such as paracetamol), or mild NSAID

- local injection of depot corticosteroids (in some cases)

- opioid-like analgesia (e.g. codeine)

- more powerful NSAIDs (frequently in combination with gastro-protective agents).

Management should include attention to independence aids, such as modified clothing, helpful household gadgets and walking aids. Patients with severe arthritis are at greater than average risk of falling and this needs consideration.

Key points

- Stick to simple analgesia

- Avoid NSAIDs

- Consider cytoprotection if NSAIDs are used

Non-steroidal anti-inflammatory drugs (NSAIDs)

NSAIDs are a potent source of serious adverse drug reactions. The most common are gastrointestinal; ibuprofen is least likely to cause bleeding, while azapropazone is most likely. Probably all old patients should be offered cytoprotection with misoprostal, H2 or proton-pump blockers. Other adverse effects are listed in Box 3.11.

Inflammatory arthropathies

Gout and pseudo-gout (pyrophosphate-arthropathy) are common and can affect any joint. They can only be diagnosed reliably by microscopy of aspirated synovial fluid. Gout is particularly common in patients with congestive heart failure and hypertension; colchicine has a special place in treatment because of the sodium-retaining properties and hypertensive effects of NSAIDs.

It is frequently difficult to decide if a patient has an inflammatory polyarthropathy of the rheumatoid type; this is partly because such patients are likely in old age to have osteoarthritis as well. A plain radiograph of the hands may reveal unsuspected current or old bone erosions typical of rheumatoid type. About 25% of 80 year olds may have low-titre false-positive tests for rheumatoid disease and systemic lupus erythematosus (SLE).

Box 3.11: Adverse effects of NSAIDs

- Oesophagitis
- Gastritis
- Ulceration at any level in the gastro-intestinal tract, which is often painless
- Interference with warfarin therapy
- Salt and water retention leading to: hypertension precipitating or exacerbating congestive heart failure
- Renal impairment reduction in glomerular filtration rate by causing afferent glomerular artery constriction
- Severe interactions with ACE inhibitors in the presence of renal artery stenosis
- Interstitial nephritis
- May worsen Parkinson's disease
- Central morphine-like action (especially with ketorolac)
- Bladder irritation and frequency

Initial management should be similar to that of osteoarthrosis above. Persistent inflammation will usually respond to around 5 mg of prednisolone per day but great care is needed to avoid long-term steroid usage due to the attendant risks. Anyone needing a higher dose, or who appears to remain steroid dependent for more than six months, should be referred for specialist advice. Treatment should be based on the clinical response rather than relying on blood tests. The erythrocyte sedimentation rate (ESR) can be expected to remain high in rheumatoid arthritis; the C-reactive protein (CRP) will reflect synovitis more accurately, and a low haemoglobin will reflect overall systemic illness.

Metabolic disorders

Hypercalcaemia

Aside from the rarities, think of hyponatraemia and hypercalcaemia in a patient with malaise

as both are relatively common. Severe hyper-calcaemia often presents with cerebral symptoms rather than constipation and polyuria. Symptomatic hypercalcaemia in older patients (as opposed to asymptomatic modest hypercalcaemia secondary to hyperparathyroidism) is almost always caused by malignancy; multiple myeloma is a common cause.

Hyponatraemia

Hyponatraemia is just as protean, more frequent, and in very old people is not usually caused by malignancy. It can be caused by fluid depletion or overload, drugs or hypothyrodism. Management may need specialist referral.

Hypernatraemia

This is also a not uncommon finding in the elderly person. It is usually caused by decreased fluid intake or increased fluid output. Failure to concentrate urine promptly in the presence of dehydration is a feature of an ageing kidney.

Diabetes mellitus

Mild failure of glucose homeostasis is very common in older people and so the range for post-prandial blood glucose is higher; it rises 0.3 mmol/l per decade of life. The mechanism of this is complex and includes insulin resistance. Most elderly diabetics are obese, and have high levels of circulating insulin (though not as high as necessary); this is the NIDDM, or type-2, diabetic syndrome. They may have relatively stable high glucose levels over long periods. During illness there is a tendency for this group to drink sugary drinks and become severely hyperglycaemic and dehydrated leading to a hyperosmolar, non-ketotic (HONK) crisis. Microvascular complications may lead to the diagnosis of NIDDM in the first place.

About 10% of elderly diabetics will develop progressive islet-cell failure (some on the basis of autoimmune destruction and detectable anti-islet-cell antibodies) which will lead to falling insulin levels and they will eventually become ketosis prone. In a series of 200 ketoacidotic emergencies analysed by the author, 40% of the

Box 3.12: Criteria for the diagnosis of diabetes mellitus and impaired glucose tolerance

	Fasting plasma glucose	Post-75 g glucose load	
		at 60 mins	at 120 mins
Diabetes			
Criterion-1	> 7.8 mmol/l on two occasions		
Criterion-2		> 11.1 mmol/l	> 11.1 mmol/l
Criterion-3			> 14 mmol/l + symptoms
Impaired			
glucose tolerance	> 7.8 mmol/l	7.8–11.1 mmol/l	

patients were over the age of 65, and half of these had been diagnosed in the previous ten years. Ketoacidosis is not common in the very old, but does carry a high mortality.

Prevalence

In areas where there is no formal screening programme, only about half the elderly diabetics are know to their GP. In the UK about 20% of the elderly population have NIDDM and another 20% impaired glucose tolerance (see Box 3.12).

Diagnosis

The renal threshold for glucose rises substantially with age so that testing the urine is not a sensitive way to pick up even severe hyperglycaemia. Standard criteria for the diagnosis with blood samples are given in Box 3.12. There is no reason why these tests cannot be done in the surgery using reagent strips providing they are repeated if the results are borderline.

The symptoms of diabetes mellitus do not really differ in old people except that nocturnal polyuria may not be noticed (because it happens anyway). Blurring of vision is common (and usually gets worse with initial treatment). Urine and perineal infections may be the only pointers.

Management

This is complex. What clearly is different from younger patients is the extra effort in education which has to be made. There is also the fear and danger of hypoglycaemia (which can present atypically with confusion rather than sweating) versus the risk of long-term complications.

Initial management is dietary. There are three steps in this:

1 estimate ideal body weight (from standard age-adjusted tables)

2 estimate target calorie intake

3 ensure balanced diet (based on calories; 55% carbohydrate, 30% fat, 15% protein).

The specialist community nurse or a general practice nurse with special responsibility for diabetic care can be of substantial help here.

Protocols for drug therapy are best developed with the local specialty group. Substances to reduce glucose absorption, e.g. biguanides and sulphonylurea all have their place. Elderly diabetics may respond promptly, and if using a sulphonylurea, choose a short-acting drug (such as tolbutamide) in the first instance to avoid hypoglycaemia; this is more likely with longer acting drugs such as glibenclamide. Control with insulin in patients who still have the capacity to regulate endogenous insulin is usually straightforward, but only if dietary intake and weight are controlled. Unless a GP has a particular interest in diabetes it would be best to have most cases periodically (perhaps every few years) reviewed by a specialist team and certainly have such a review involving a specialist diabetic nurse if a transfer to insulin is contemplated.

The patient should be regularly reviewed in the community for control (using glycated haemoglobin measurement if possible) and checked for complications. Lens opacities make accurate examination of the optic fundi difficult. It is wise to have vision and the fundi checked by an expert at the outset because of the high incidence of early complications, and afterwards every five years.

Frail patients and diabetes

With very elderly and frail patients it may be appropriate to opt for purely symptomatic control, and not aim to prevent microvascular complications. It is thought that infection is more likely if the plasma glucose is persistently above 12 mmol/l, probably because of glycation of white blood cells, but nevertheless, many patients find it difficult to keep glucose levels below this. It is difficult to expect a change in a life-long intake of sugar and there are circumstances in which it is unreasonable and inappropriate to expect this.

Key points

- Diagnosis is often late
- Spend more time on patient education
- Beware of hypoglycaemia
- Avoid long acting drugs
- Regular specialist assessment of vision is important

Thyroid disorders

Prevalence

Thyroid dysfunction is relatively common in the old: hypothyroidism is present in upwards of 5% (mainly females) of the over 65s, and hyperthyroidism in around 1–2%. Modern biochemical tests are not expensive and are very powerful in distinguishing normal function from either under- or over-activity and treatment is normally simple and leads to major clinical improvements.

Diagnosis

Hyperthyroidism characteristically does not present with over-activity, although weight loss and a tachycardia at rest may be present. Sometimes,

the only manifestation is cardiac. Atrial fibrillation is very common in the old (> 5% total elderly population) and may be the result of thyroid over-activity. Apathetic thyrotoxicosis is well described in the literature but is not common. By contrast, the cerebral consequences of hypothyroidism are said to be excitation and myxoedema madness.

The other mode of presentation of hypothyroidism to stress, apart from those emphasized in the standard texts, is its effects on sodium and water balance in the old. In the hypothyroid state, the body has a problem handling a sodium load, and in excreting free water. So depending on the salt and water intake, subjects may be oedematous, hyponatraemic or both. Indeed, unexplained isolated pleural or pericardial effusions (with normal cardiac function and no pulmonary pathology) and unexplained ascites with or without facial and peripheral oedema may result from hypothyroidism. Therefore thyroid function should always be checked in a hyponatraemic patient.

Key points

- Have a low threshold for measuring thyroid function
- Thyroid function tests are indicated in all cases of atrial fibrillation, hyponatraemia, and in most cases of heart failure
- Treat myxoedema cautiously (high incidence of associated ischaemic heart disease)

Pituitary dysfunction

More cases are coming to light with more widespread use of hormonal assays and cranial scanning. Hypothalamic lesions may present as lack of thirst, failure of blood pressure and temperature control. Pan-hypopituitaryism is of very slow onset and presents with weakness, loss of libido and secondary sexual characteristics and skin pallor, and later by hypotension, hyponatraemia and occasionally hypoglycaemia. The finding of a low thyroxine with a normal or low thyroid stimulating hormone (TSH) measurement should point to further assessment of the pituitary except in an acutely ill patient in whom the 'sick euthyroid' syndrome is more likely. Paradoxically, low follicle stimulating hormone (FSH) and luteinizing hormone (LH) in a post-menopausal female are similar pointers. Even mild adrenocorticotropic hormone (ACTH) deficiency (that is with normal basal and stimulated levels or circulating cortisol) can cause malaise and hyponatraemia when the patient is ill or stressed.

Osteoporosis

Prevalence

Probably all current 80 year old females could be regarded as suffering from osteoporosis (OP) to the extent that they are more at risk of fractures. Prevalence in men is about a tenth of that in females. This is a major issue for primary care and the health services generally with OP accounting for a substantial proportion of wrist, hip and vertebral fractures, and much morbidity.

Diagnosis

Early in the disease, formal assessment of bone mass using a densitometer is the only reliable current method. Later, plain X-rays, especially of the spine and hips can provide semi-quantitative evidence (especially examining the trabecular lines in the hips). Finally, in the late stages, vertebral collapse with kyphosis (the dowager's hump) become obvious.

Painful vertebral collapse in the female is usually due to osteoporosis but cancer and myeloma should not be forgotten. A good physical examination should include a detailed examination of the breast of a woman, and the prostate in a man. A plain chest radiograph, and lateral radiographs of the appropriate area of the spine will usually settle the matter. A measurement of prostatic-specific antigen (in a male) will usually be helpful if secondary cancer is a serious possibility, and the possibility of bone infection (especially in a male where the distribution tends to be the same as that of prostatic secondaries) should not be ignored.

Various factors worth consideration in osteoporosis are the age of menopause and whether there has been an oophorectomy (previously a common accompaniment of a hysterectomy). Calcium and vitamin deficiency may well be important factors in bone loss, especially in older people. A dietary and gastrointestinal history (for malabsorption) are therefore important. Cigarette smoking is thought to have a significant impact on vertebral bone, and excessive alcohol consumption has an adverse effect. In males, who are less prone to symptomatic osteoporosis than females, testosterone deficiency should be considered in the younger age groups, and in both sexes the possibility of hypo-pituitaryism considered. Conversely, cortisol excess is a well recognized cause of bone wasting and exogenous corticosteroids are a major factor. Other causes include hyperthyroidism, immobilization and chronic renal failure.

Management

In the peri-menopausal period, dietary supplementation of calcium and hormone replacement therapy are standard treatment. Fluoride therapy has recently been shown to reduce fracture rates as well as increase bone mass (there had previously been some doubt about this because of the toxic effects of fluoride in higher doses). Bisphosphonates can reduce the fracture rate in all cases.

Age-associated osteoporosis is treated by calcium (1–1.5 g/day) and vitamin-D (400 IU/day) supplementation. One pint of milk (full-fat or skimmed) contains about 750 mg of elemental calcium, and for those on an otherwise good diet this may be adequate. Fish and cod liver oil contain vitamin-D, which some anti-medicine minded patients can be persuaded to take. Anyone in the UK who does not go out in the sun regularly will have low blood vitamin-D levels, and during the winter and spring many old people are partially deficient. This is a particular risk in nursing homes in which a case can be made for routine administration of vitamin-D.

All types of osteoporosis can be improved by oral bisphosphonates. They must be taken on a calcium-free stomach (i.e. fasting) and this makes compliance difficult. They are expensive and current drugs can have unpleasant gastrointestinal side-effects.

Movement disorders

Extra-pyramidal defects and Parkinson's disease

Idiopathic Parkinson's disease (IPD, see below) is present in about 2% of the elderly population. The signs include poverty of facial and other movements, tremor (see below) and various forms of increased muscle tone. Minor degrees of increased tone are best brought out by asking the patient to perform a simple unstressed movement of the contralateral side; such as gently opening and closing the hand. Cogwheeling is probably always abnormal but is not diagnostic of Parkinson's disease. Rating scales, such as Webster's scale provide a useful checklist of items relevant to the diagnosis of Parkinson's disease, as well as providing a means of monitoring progress and treatment. Patients in their 80s rarely present with classical IPD. There is a tendency for gait to be more affected and bradykinesia to be more prominent than tremor. Other neurological signs and the presence of primitive reflexes point to more extensive CNS disease. When assessing mental function it is important to give the subject adequate time to respond as thoughts and their expression may be slowed in a similar manner to their movements. Other conditions causing extra-pyramidal features are common, such as vascular Parkinson's disease, progressive supra nuclear palsy (Steele Richardson Syndrome) and the Shy Drager Syndrome, all of which respond poorly to L-dopa, and normal-pressure hydrocephalus, which may respond to shunting.

Treatment

All drugs effective in Parkinson's disease have significant side-effects. The most notable of these are confusion, hallucinations, orthostatic hypotension and constipation. It is therefore very important to have a good reason for treating someone with an extra-pyramidal defect, and to have an objective means for deciding whether there has been a significant response or not, such as a timed ten-metre walk and a measured repetitive task for assessing hand function. These are then repeated one hour after 100 mg of L-dopa (as Sinemet or Madopar). If there is no clear improvement, patients are treated for two weeks and the measures repeated. The main principle with older patients is to use the lowest effective dose. Normally patients are happy to take small doses frequently, but an alternative to avoid fluctuations is to employ a long-acting agent with perhaps an initial short-acting dose in the morning.

Other therapy includes adaptations in the home, alterations to clothing and physiotherapy. These can be very important as frail people often have major adverse effects from anti-Parkinson drugs.

Other drugs and side-effects

L-dopa commonly causes nausea, hallucinations, confusion, severe orthostatic hypotension and constipation. Nausea can be countered by giving small more frequent doses and adding the dopa antagonist domperidone (which only seems to penetrate the brain stem). Hallucinations may be controlled by small doses and by avoiding L-dopa soon before bedtime. It is wise to check a mental test score before and after initiating therapy in frail patients, and to check lying and standing blood pressure in all. When the equivalent of 600 mg of L-dopa per day (given in 62.5 mg increments or in a sustained release formulation) is not proving effective control, it is time for a specialist referral. Tremor is more likely to respond to an anti-cholinergic such as benzhexol 1 mg once or twice daily, but be on the look out for hallucinations and confusion. Nevertheless, some patients require and can be maintained on L-dopa and an anti-cholinergic to great benefit.

Tremor

Tremor in old age can be very difficult to sort out. Titubation of the head and oro-facial dyskinesia are fairly characteristic, as is the classical pill-rolling tremor of Parkinson's disease. One common problem is simply to equate tremor with Parkinson's disease and therefore inappropriately prescribe L-dopa.

Senile tremor is unlikely to respond to drugs but as it is mainly an action tremor (which is quite the reverse of a Parkinsonian tremor) it can cause great disability as well as embarrassment. Often there is a family history and it can improve with alcohol. The following drugs may be tried for a serious non-Parkinson, non-cerebellar tremor: the centrally acting beta-blocker, propranolol; sodium valproate (even though it causes tremor in overdosage); and the dopamine depleter tetrabenazine. All should be given cautiously and patients monitored carefully.

Mention should be made of the severe consequences of dyskinesia secondary to Phenothiazine and other neuroleptic use. It can be very disabling, and unlike in younger patients, may occur after just one dose of chlorpromazine. Therefore neuroleptics should be used with caution and only for good reason in the elderly. It is the author's practice to avoid chlorpromazine (which additionally often produces troublesome orthostatic hypotension) but there are no controlled data, and all major tranquillizers should be regarded as suspect in this regard. Neither is malignant neuroleptic syndrome rare and it carries an appreciable mortality. Thioridazine possibly has a lower incidence of extra-pyramidal effects than chlorpromazine. Tremor due to phenothiazine should be treated, if possibly by withdrawal of the drug but this is not always successful. L-dopa is of no value in this situation.

Key points

- Not all tremor is due to Parkinson's disease

- Measure the response to therapy objectively

- Use small doses of L-dopa or a long-acting preparation

- Avoid chlorpromazine

Aches and pains

Polymyalgia rheumatica, giant cell arteritis and related conditions

Generalized aches and pains must be one of the banes of the primary care physician's life. Polymyalgia rheumatica (PMR) and giant cell arteritis (GCA) appear to be so common that it is worth asking specific questions relating to these two conditions.

Polymyalgia rheumatica (PMR)

Polymyalgia rheumatica is a condition with generalized aches and pains and evidence of a chronic inflammatory disorder with elevated acute-phase proteins and usually some suppression of haemoglobin production. Clinical features, which are diagnostically helpful, are early difficulty in getting the arms above the head or combing the hair. Patients may have some (understandable) difficulty in reconciling their symptoms with the lack of tenderness in their muscles and will comment on the difficulty in deciding where the pain comes from. The pain is usually around the upper or lower limb girdle but is often difficult to localize. If the muscles are tender polymyositis is more likely, and stiffness may be more prominent than pain. Polymyalgia rheumatica may be insidious in onset and wax and wane, and can exist for many years off and on. A mild mono- or poly-arthropathy is not rare in PMR and GCA and may precede more typical symptoms. Just to confuse matters, acute and sub-acute seronegative polyarthritis is by no means rare in the eighth decade and be beware of the high incidence of 'falsely' positive anti-nuclear antibodies and rheumatoid factors in older people.

Incidence

As neither PMR nor GCA have clear-cut diagnostic criteria accurate incidence and prevalence figures are not available. These disorders are almost unheard of below the age of 50 years and the annual incidence rises steeply over the age of 60 and may be as high as 4 in 1000 elderly in the UK; a practitioner may expect to see about one new case a year.

Diagnostic tests

Complaints of aches and pains are a good indication to measure the haemoglobin, CRP and ESR; in most significant inflammatory disorders one or more will be abnormal. It may also be worth measuring the creatinine phosphokinase, although true myositis is much less common than PMR. In PMR the haemoglobin is almost invariably on the low side, if not frankly abnormal, the platelet count is often elevated and the total white cell count may be slightly elevated (say up to $14 \times 10^9/l$). The serum alkaline phosphatase is often also slightly elevated, and one should expect the alpha$_1$-acid glycoprotein and other acute-phase proteins to remain chronically elevated. A significant abnormality in the immunoglobulins strongly suggests some other disorder.

The differential diagnosis includes other causes of the pains and weakness, and other causes of raised inflammatory indices. A high white-cell count, and high IgM or IgG suggest infection such as in the urine or chest.

Therapy

In PMR initial therapy is also an important diagnostic aid; there is probably no other condition which responds so promptly to 7.5 or 10 mg of prednisolone per day. While it is the case that some need a relatively high dose of steroid for complete suppression, high-dose steroid will make even infected patients feel well for a while. It is therefore best to start with the lowest effective dose. With PMR subsequent doses should depend on symptoms rather than the inflammatory markers which may require a much higher dose to suppress fully, despite the patient feeling well.

Giant cell arteritis

Giant cell arteritis is a vasculitis which affects medium sized arteries throughout the body. It often starts with PMR-like symptoms but headaches, scalp tenderness and jaw claudication suggest localized ischaemia and are helpful when present. Occasionally patients just present with ill-health and the diagnosis is only made after histological examination of an artery biopsied at the end of a long fruitless diagnostic work-up. The inflammatory markers are almost always very high but as biopsy proven GCA with normal (or relatively normal) inflammatory indices does exist, giving advice on how far to pursue symptomatic patients with normal blood tests is not easy. Perhaps the best strategy when in doubt is watchful waiting; although if GCA is a serious possibility then urgent treatment or specialist referral is indicated.

The condition seems to have a predilection for the posterior ciliary branches of the ophthalmic arteries which on account of their small size may thrombose leading to acute ischaemic optic neuropathy and permanent blindness. It is this dreaded complication that prompts emergency investigation and treatment of an elderly patient with new headache and localized scalp tenderness.

Treatment

Most authorities consider that unlike PMR, GCA should be treated promptly with high-dose corticosteroid (say prednisolone 60 mg/day in a robust subject) and subsequent steroid doses determined by regular monitoring of the inflammatory indices. While PMR should ordinarily be a community diagnosed and managed condition, patients with suspected GCA should be referred for specialist assessment even if started on therapy before referral. Old people frequently suffer adverse events from high-dose corticosteroids, with hypertension, heart failure and severe osteoporosis being common. It is the author's current practice to consider early addition of immunosuppressive agents, such as azathioprine or Methotrexate, in severe cases and to use dexamethasone in those exhibiting significant salt retention. All patients are given some prophylaxis for osteoporosis as vertebral fractures during therapy are all too common.

Key points

- Giant cell arteritis can be a medical emergency – beware ophthalmic complications

- Adverse effects for corticosteroids in the old are very high

- Treat polymyalgia on symptoms

- With aches and pains check the blood count, ESR and CRP

- Think of osteoporosis prophylaxis in patients on long-term steroids

Generalized aches and pains

So many disorders can present with mysterious pains that it is hard to give a sensible analysis. For example, one series of older patients with bacterial endocarditis revealed backache as one of the commonest early features. A normal haemoglobin, CRP and ESR go a long way to ruling-out a serious constitutional inflammatory process. One worry is systemic lupus erythematosus (SLE) and various other vasculitides which may be present even when these tests are normal. When the cause of generalized symptoms is not clear, watchful-waiting with repeat tests may be the best policy.

Cancer is common in old age and may underline many mysterious complaints. The watchful part of waiting should include measuring weight. The physical examination should be sufficiently sensitive to pick up extensive prostate or breast cancer, and myeloma is easy to exclude with the above blood tests and a urine sample for light chains. A chest radiograph may well reveal a variety of tumours when they are widespread. Consider myositis with osteomalacia. Most patients will have non-specific aches and malaise rather than the classic descriptions in standard textbooks.

Skin ulceration and pressure sores

Pressure sores

Definition

Pressure sores result from infarction of the skin and/or underlying tissues. They vary from loss of the epidermis only, to deep lesions penetrating as far as bone. Treating a deep pressure sore can be very costly.

Prevalence

Pressure sores used to be quite uncommon in domiciliary practice. With more dependent people being cared for at home, and with the greater involvement of GPs in managing sick patients and in nursing homes, a clear understanding of the causes and prevention of pressure sores has become very important. No age is immune, but in practice serious sores are mostly found in the elderly. Good geriatric units use continuous monitoring of their pressure-sore rates as a form of quality assessment.

Pathology

Ischaemia occurs if the surface pressure exceeds that in the arteriolar end of skin capillaries (about 30 mmHg). Ischaemia also occurs if the skin is longitudinally deformed (shear stress) as this deforms the capillary loops which run at right angles to the skin surface. In a healthy subject, the skin and underlying tissues may survive as long as six to eight hours ischaemia, but in a subject with a poor blood supply (e.g. as a result of heart failure, dehydration, or vascular sclerosis) or poor oxygen supply (e.g. as a result of anaemia, hypoxia, or tissue oedema), the period of ischaemia which the skin and dermis will survive is much less and may be as low as two hours. The worst sores that the author has seen have occurred in either very dehydrated or septicaemic patients in whom multiple defects are probably involved (see Box 3.13).

It is recognized that there is a time/pressure relationship in the development of ulcers, and that moderate excess pressure over a prolonged

Box 3.13: Factors relevant to pressure sores

- Mechanical factors
  - pressure
  - shearing
  - maceration (can increase shear)

- Movement disorders
  - paralysis
  - stupor and coma (including drug-induced)
  - bradykinesia (parkinsonism)

- Cellular hypoxia and other factors
  - oedema
  - anaemia
  - systemic hypoxia
  - heart failure
  - dehydration

- Neuropathy
  - diabetes
  - alcoholism

- Poor nutritional status

Box 3.14: The Norton Scale of pressure-sore risk

Physical condition	
good	4
fair	3
poor	2
very bad	1
Mental state	
alert	4
apathetic	3
confused	2
stupor	1
Activity	
ambulant	4
walk with 1	3
chairbound	2
bedbound	1
Mobility	
full	4
limited	3
very limited	2
immobile	1
Incontinence	
none	4
occasional	3
usually	2
doubly	1
<12 HIGH RISK, 12–14 ABOVE AVERAGE RISK	

This scale is suggested because it is easy to remember, quick to do and is well validated. More complex scales are sometimes used by nurses and in hospital.

period may lead to as bad ulceration as shorter periods of intense pressure. Underlying tissues may be more susceptible to infarction than the epidermis itself, and the lesion may start with underlying necrosis followed by later ulceration of the skin. In this way the injury does not present for a day or so.

For a patient lying on a standard UK hospital bed, the sacrum, hips and heels are subject to pressure well in excess (possibly double) of the 30 mmHg tolerable level; beds at home tend to be more forgiving. However, there is much more friction between a wet sheet and skin, than a dry sheet, so the elderly subject propped up in bed on wet sheets, and using their heels to lever themselves up as they slide down, is liable to shear damage to the sacrum and heels. Heels are

also prone to ischaemia when incorrectly placed on wheelchair leg-rests, or stuck over the footboard of a bed. It is important to include the risk of pressure sores in your overall assessment of a patient (see Box 3.14).

In the home, pressure sores are not common. There may be several reasons: relevant factors may be the softness of domestic beds, and the relative fitness of patients compared with the sickest patients in hospital. Informal carers are often very adept at moving a subject they know very well, and may give better care than is initially given to patients in emergency facilities, or when formal but not very experienced carers are substituted for a long-standing informal carer.

Pressure sore sites

The hip, sacrum and heels are the most common sites to be involved; the latter are especially troublesome as this often interferes with mobility for long periods. Almost any area of the body can be affected, especially following a fall and pressure at unusual sites, for example skin necrosis over a gibus. Drug overdose, age and subsequent immobility can be associated with skin ischaemia even in young subjects.

Pressure sores should be treated with the following principles in mind:

- relieve the pressure (regular two-hourly turning is almost guaranteed to do this)

- resolve overt local infection

- remove large areas of necrotic tissue as this may harbour unnoticed infection and delay healing

- keep the ulcerated areas as moist as possible (as this is known to promote granulation tissue)

- keep dressing changes to the minimum compatible with clean ulcers (as each removal is likely to remove granulation tissue)

- avoid topical agents where possible as these are commonly toxic to granulation tissue and allergy may develop, as is common with varicose ulcers

- treat significant systemic disorders (especially anaemia)

- attend to general nutrition (bearing in mind that patients with significant ulcers are often catabolic and may have difficulty maintaining nitrogen balance).

Also bear in mind that anyone with an ulcerated lesion is more prone to bacteraemic or septi-caemic illness.

Prevention

Nowhere is the maxim 'prevention better than cure' more apposite; just a few hours inappro-priate care can lead to weeks or months of intensive therapy and the need for an expensive pressure-relieving mattress in the home. The most important point is recognizing risk (see Box 3.14). Moving the patient's position religiously every two hours will almost guarantee freedom from necrosis but this is often difficult to achieve in practice, especially at night. Few pressure-relieving devices are guaranteed to keep skin pressure below 30 mmHg and should therefore be regarded as a means to reduce the frequency of turning, rather than abolishing the need for turning.

Key points

- Pressure sores are usually a sign of poor care
- For effective prevention and therapy you must work effectively with the nursing team
- There are no magic cures or medic-aments
- Bear in mind the high risk older people
  - those with heart failure, hypoxia and arterio-sclerosis
  - those with anaemia, CHF or tissue oedema
  - the immobile and especially the bed-bound
  - those in hospital

Lower-limb skin ulceration

With skin ulcers on the lower limb, varicose and ischaemic ulcers must be considered, and at any site a large lesion of pyoderma gangrenosum may, initially, be thought to result from pressure. Venous ulcers are normally sited at a charac-teristic position on the inner aspect of the lower calf, with evidence of previous venous insuf-ficiency. They often have a bleeding edge and healthy tissue in the centre. The high prevalence of venous ulceration in the old should be a spur to the use of adequate therapy and limb compression for venous disorders in younger patients.

Arterial ulcers usually occur in the extremities and there are usually poor or absent peripheral pulses. Ulceration often results from both arterial and venous insufficiency so that specialist advice may be necessary. Doppler studies are now mandatory if there is any doubt about arterial or venous causation. Neuropathic ulcers should be considered, e.g. in diabetes or alcoholism.

An additional point to consider is that the skin on older legs is often very thin, especially in pa-tients who have received corticosteroid therapy, and may easily be removed, like a de-gloving injury, by relatively minor trauma.

The context, site and characteristics of the lesion in each case usually make the diagnosis fairly clear.

Treatment

The main therapy for varicose ulceration is elevation and pressure bandaging. Older limbs are frequently ischaemic and pressure bandaging is problematic when arterial insufficiency is present, and in these circumstances controlled-pressure bandaging with simultaneous Doppler measurements of the arterial pulse may be nec-essary. Pressure bandages with inbuilt pressure graduations are available and make application by relatively junior staff safer. Pure arterial ulcers will normally mandate specialist referral.

Syncope

Syncope arises from either a sudden interruption of adequate blood supply to the brain stem, or in the normal electrical activity of the brain (as in a generalized tonic clonic seizure). Various fac-tors operate in older people to make them more sensitive to alterations in cerebral perfusion. For example, atherosclerotic cerebral arteries and hypertension reduce cerebrovascular autoreg-ulation and narrowing of larger vessels increases the adverse effect of lowering mean central (i.e. aortic) blood pressure. Thus, modest falls in blood pressure of older people can have a dramatic effect.

Unconsciousness caused by hypotension is almost always heralded by an aura of impending collapse. An older patient may just report this feeling as 'giddiness', or, more commonly, will forget it altogether after the subsequent uncon-sciousness, thus a valuable piece of diagnostic information is lost. Presumably this failure to report is due to a greater effect of the subsequent cerebral ischaemia on the older brain.

Unconsciousness caused by a cerebral dysrhythmia is difficult to detect unless witnessed because elderly patients are often confused for some time afterwards. True unconsciousness (as opposed to pre-syncope, or the feeling of impending unconsciousness) is usually due to either a cerebral or cardiac dysrhythmia, or a fit secondary to sudden severe hypotension.

Investigation

All patients should have a resting 12-lead ECG and several blood pressure measurements in different circumstances such as lying and standing. 24 hours ECG monitoring, or fitting a cardiomemo type device is reasonable depend-ing on the circumstances. Totally unprovoked unconsciousness in someone with pre-existing cardiac disease is very likely to be due to a dysrhythmia (see page 48). Usually after a single attack it is most helpful to discuss potential aetiology with the patient, spouse or others close to the patient, and to try and obtain a detailed description of any subsequent attack, including a measure of the carotid pulse (after you have checked for hypersensitivity). Do not request an EEG without specialist advice as they are very difficult to interpret in the old. Finding a sig-nificant cranial abnormality on cranial computer-ized tomography (CT) or magnetic resonance imaging (MRI) raises the prior probability of seizure substantially and is therefore, similar to knowing there is severe cardiac disease, diag-nostically useful. Patients with both cardiac and cerebral disease are problematic.

Key points

- Unconsciousness always has a cause

- A witness is often more helpful than multiple tests

- EEGs are frequently abnormal in the old, and are therefore often not diagnostic-ally helpful

- A cranial CT or MRI may be less sensit-ive but more specific in leading to a diagnosis

Hypotension

Older people have more variable blood pressure and are more prone to episodic hypotension and orthostatic hypotension (see Box 3.15). Ortho-static hypotension is quite variable and is often difficult to demonstrate. The blood pressure should be taken lying, and then immediately on rising detecting the change in pulse volume at the brachial or radial artery. It is not unusual for the blood pressure to drop temporarily on standing, and then rise to normal or above normal levels

Box 3.15: Factors relevant to orthostatic hypotension

- Antihypertensive agents

- Anti-Parkinsonian agents

- Most antidepressants, especially tricy-clic agents

- Most neuroleptics

- Diuretic-induced hypovolaemia

- Relative 'hypovolaemia' induced by large capacity varicose veins

- Hypokalaemia, the mechanism is possibly via aggravating the effect of autonomic neuropathy

- Early-morning hypovolaemia, especi-ally with nocturnal polyuria

within a minute or so. Conversely, it may be normal immediately on standing and only fall after a couple of minutes of standing still. Finally, some people suffer from exertional hypotension. This may be particularly true of those with significant aortic stenosis and those on anti-hypertensives (perhaps particularly beta-blockers if the pulse rate does not rise on exercise). This is best demonstrated by taking the blood pressure again after a significant period of exercise. Alternatively, a 24-hour blood pressure monitor may pick up serious fluctuations in everyday life.

Key points

- Think of low blood pressure as a cause of malaise and unwillingness to rise

- Bear aortic stenosis in mind

- Many drugs cause severe orthostatic hypotension

Disturbances in cardiac rhythm

Tachycardia

Disturbances in cardiac rhythm are common, even the norm, in old age. Fibrosis of conducting tracts in the atria leads to atrial arrhythmias and atrial fibrillation, and fibrosis or calcification of the conducting tracts in the intraventricular septum may lead to various degrees of heart block.[10] About 5% of the population aged over 75 years have atrial fibrillation, and these subjects have a substantial increase in overall mortality and up to a five-fold increase in stroke incidence.

Determined efforts should be made to convert recent onset atrial fibrillation into sinus rhythm because not only is the need for anticoagulation removed but exercise tolerance is improved. Established stable atrial fibrillation resistant to chemical or electrical cardioversion should normally be controlled with digoxin, and the risk of atrial thrombosis reduced by warfarin (INR

2.0–3.0) or aspirin. Paroxysmal atrial fibrillation or exercise-induced tachycardia are usually poorly controlled by digoxin, and a beta-blocker (such as sotalol) or a calcium-channel blocker (such as verapamil) or amiodarone should be used either alone or with digoxin to achieve control. All patients with atrial fibrillation should have thyroid function measured, as thyrotoxicosis is readily treated. Patients on amiodarone will need regular thyroid function tests (request a TSH measurement not a T4), and an intermittent lung function test, or a chest X-ray, to pick up pulmonary fibrosis. All will get corneal deposits which may interfere with night vision. Some patients with variable atrial rates (such as in the sick-sinus syndrome) need a pacemaker and an anti-dysrhythmic agent.

Key points

- With atrial fibrillation think about cardioversion

- The elderly (stiff) heart is more in need of atrial systole than the young heart

- Atrial tachycardias rarely cause blackouts

Tachy-arrhythmias in a fit population aged 65 years and over without coronary artery disease

- atrial fibrillation   5%
- isolated ventricular extrasystoles   80%
- frequent ventricular ectopics   17%
- frequent supra-ventricular ectopics   26%
- paroxysmal atrial tachycardia   13%
- non-sustained ventricular tachycardia   4%

Bradycardias

Alteration to the atrial conduction tissues also leads to bradycardias, sino-atrial block and the sick-sinus syndrome. Fibrosis of the atrioven-tricular-node and conducting tracts also leads to heart block. Calcific aortic stenosis may also lead to heart block as may myocardial ischaemia and infarction. Digoxin may well precipitate heart block in these patients. About 60% of all permanent pacemakers are implanted in patients aged over 70 years: roughly half are implanted for heart block and half for the sick-sinus syndrome. Be aware that patients with a long PR-interval and left-axis deviation on their plain ECGs are prone to heart block if given drugs which interfere with conduction in the heart (such as digoxin, beta-blockers and most calcium-channel blockers).

Key points

- With bradycardia, review the prescription sheet

- Beware of using drugs that slow atrio-ventricular conduction

---

Falls

Prevalence

Injuries sustained in falling are a major cause of morbidity and mortality in the old. In 85 year olds, the annual death rate from falling is about 150 per 100 000. About a third of 80 year olds will admit to 'falling', but possibly the majority have at least one potentially serious trip or stumble every year. Heavy drinkers probably under-report when they fall – perhaps out of a wish to deny or conceal the problem.

Aetiology and differential diagnosis

Some of the factors predisposing to falls are given in Box 3.16, while significant points in the history and examination are listed in Box 3.17.

It may be helpful to distinguish falling over from the legs giving way; the latter is so characteristic that it is worth specific mention. Patients who have fallen almost always say they have tripped, but when prompted may agree that

their fall was 'like my knee being hit from behind'. This happens quite suddenly, for no obvious reason (unlike a fall in a neurologically impaired patient induced by turning or negotiat-ing an obstacle) and the patient crumples down, rather than falling over. If help is at hand, the patient can rise and walk immediately. There is no giddiness (though this may be spuriously reported and should be analysed carefully), no loss or impairment of consciousness, no paralysis or neurological symptoms, no pain and usually no serious injury. In the author's experience, once this story is elicited, there is little point in further investigation and management should be dir-ected to improving the safety of the environment for example by the provision of an appropriate alarm. The hip may also spontaneously fracture and the patient fall secondary to this.

The other factor in the presentation of falls which should be emphasized is the importance of reviewing the prescription. Mention of alcohol has already been made, but several drugs, notably hypnotics, have been implicated in falls. It is repeated several times that drugs can pro-voke almost any illness or syndrome, and that as older people take so much medication it is hardly surprising that drugs are so frequently implicated as the major, or aggravating, factor in many illnesses. Falls are no exception.

Box 3.16: Predisposing factors to falls

Extrinsic

- Lighting, low or uneven illumination
- Bed and chair heights
- Low cupboards and switches, falling forward on bending down is common
- Uneven or slippery surfaces, any surface on which a toe can catch can be hazardous, including long-pile carpets
- Stairs and steps, especially those that are not railed or that have uneven step caps
- Baths

Intrinsic

- CNS disturbances, increased body sway (which is a normal accompaniment of ageing); poor righting reflexes, reaction times and sensory disturbances; poor balance: vestibular, brain-stem dysfunction and cerebellar disease
- various CNS diseases, especially stroke, Parkinson's disease, late dementia, and drug effects
- Poor vision
- Any cause of unconsciousness
- Myoclonic jerks
- Muscular weakness, especially affecting the lower limbs
- Joint instability, especially of knees and ankles
- Sudden fall in blood pressure (see Box 3.18)

Box 3.17: Falls and older patients

- Some points in the history
    - falling over versus legs giving way
    - loss of consciousness, remembers falling?
    - the specific circumstances of the fall or falls, which may only be evident on visiting the home
    - recent use or alteration of a drug?
- Some points in the examination
    - muscular strength, especially at ankles and quads
    - joint deformities and instability, especially knees and ankles
    - significant neurological deficits, especially stroke, Parkinsonism, neuropathy, and consider gait dyspraxia such as in advanced Alzheimer's disease
    - Blood pressure lying, standing (immediate), standing (1 minute) after exertion

Box 3.18: Some causes of a sudden fall in blood pressure relevant to older patients

- Autonomic neuropathy

- Varicose veins, leading to increased venous pooling on standing

- Postprandial hypotension

- Hypotension after a hot bath

- Drug-induced vasodilatation, e.g. nitrates for angina, anti-hypertensives and anti-cholinergics

- Nocturnal polyuria with morning hypovolaemia

- Diuretic-induced hypovolaemia, mid-morning especially in combination with other hypotensive agents such as ACE inhibitors

- Exercise-induced vasodilation, especially in the presence of aortic stenosis

- Vasodepressor (vagal) syncope

- Carotid sinus hypersensitivity, falls or symptoms on turning or pressing on the neck

- Bradycardia (relative) on exercise, e.g. beta-adrenoreceptor blockers, or in sino-atrial disease

- Paroxysmal rapid atrial fibrillation, in the presence of increased left ventricular stiffness

References

1 Fairweather DS and Evans JG (1990) Ageing, in *The Metabolic and Molecular Basis of Acquired Disease* (eds Cohen RD, Alberti KGMM, Lewis B, Denman AM). Baillière Tindall, Eastbourne, pp. 213–36.

2 European Working Party on High Blood Pressure in the Elderly (EWPHE) (1985) Mortality and morbidity results from the European Working Party on High Blood Pressure in the Elderly trial. *Lancet* i:1349–54.

3 Launer LJ, Masaki K, Petrovitch H *et al.* (1995) The association between midlife blood pressure levels and late-life cognitive function: the Honolulu-Asia study. *J American Medical Association* **274**:1846, 1851.

4 SHEP Cooperative Research Group (1991) Prevention of stroke by anti-hypertensive drug treatment in older persons with isolated systolic hypertension. Final results of the systolic hypertension program (SHEP). *J American Medical Association* **265**:2256–64.

5 Lakatta EG and Gerstenblith G (1992) Cardiovascular disorders, in *Oxford Textbook of Geriatric Medicine* (eds Grimley Evans J, Williams TF). Oxford University Press, Oxford.

6 Dennis M and Warlow C (1991) Strategy for stroke. *BMJ* **303**:636–8.

7 Sheldon JH (1963) The effect of age on the control of sway. *Gerontologia Clinica* **5**:129–38.

8 Fox RH, Woodward PM, Exton-Smith AN *et al.* (1973) Body temperature in the elderly: a national study of physiological, social and environmental conditions. *BMJ* i:200–6.

9 Brocklehurst JC (1985) The genitourinary system, in *Textbook of Geriatric Medicine and Gerontology* (eds Brocklehurst JC, Tallis RC, Fillit HM), 3rd edn. Churchill Livingstone, Edinburgh.

10 Fairweather DS (1992) Aging of the heart and cardiovascular system. *Reviews in Clinical Gerontology* **2**:83–103.

Further reading

Abrams WB and Berkow R (eds) (1990) *The Merck Manual of Geriatrics*. Merck Sharp & Dhome Research Laboratories, New Jersey, USA.

Brocklehurst JC and Tallis RC (eds) (1992) *Textbook of Geriatric Medicine and Gerontology,* 4th edn. Churchill Livingstone, Edinburgh.

Fairweather DS (1991) Delirium, in *Psychiatry in the Elderly* (eds Jacoby R and Oppenheimer C). Oxford University Press, Oxford.

Fairweather DS and Campbell AJ (1991) Diagnostic accuracy: the effects of multiple aetiology and the degradation of information in old age. *J Roy Coll Phys* **25**:105–10.

Grimley Evans J and Williams TF (eds) (1992) *Oxford Textbook of Geriatric Medicine.* Oxford University Press, Oxford.

Henry D *et al.* (1996) Variability in risk of gastrointestinal complications from non-steroidal anti-inflammatory drugs: a meta-analysis. *BMJ* **312**:1563–6.

Nordin BEC *et al.* (1993) Osteoporosis, in *Metabolic Bone and Stone Disease* (eds Nordin BEC, Need AG and Morris HA), 3rd edn. Churchill Livingstone, Edinburgh.

Pajk M (1990) Pressure sores, in *The Merck Manual of Geriatrics* (eds Abrams WB and Berkow R), Merck Sharp & Dhome Research Laboratories, New Jersey, USA.

Appendix: Alterations in routine laboratory tests with age

Hb
11.5–17 g/dl (males and females)
The lower limit of normal is the same in young and old, although there are fewer older subjects with high Hb levels

WBC
$3.0–9.0 \times 10^9/l$
A slight reduction in the frail old, and a decreased recruitment during infection

ESR
5–30 mm/hr
Slight polyclonal elevation in the IgG (see globulins below) and slight reduction in albumin (below) may cause some elevation to the 'normal' ESR. If the globulins and albumin are well within the normal range, then the ESR should be in the normal range for younger subjects as well

CRP
< 8 mg/l
Unchanged in old age

Albumin
33–49 g/l
A slight reduction with age

Globulins (total)
20–41 g/l
A significant increase with age

Sodium
135–145 mmol/l
The range is slightly lower if (stable) patients are included in the reference population. Levels below 130 mmol/l should be considered as significant, but patients with levels between 130 and 134 mmol/l are probably at risk from significant hyponatraemia when ill

Potassium
3.6–5.2 mmol/l
Reference ranges are slightly wider in old age

Calcium
males 2.19–2.59 mmol/l
females 2.18–2.68 mmol/l
Modest elevation not rare in elderly females (usually associated with detectable levels of parathyroid hormone) and usually asymptomatic

Phosphate   males 0.66–1.27 mmol/l
females 0.94–1.56 mmol/l
Levels are raised in older females but unchanged in older males

Alkaline   22–82 iu/l
phosphatase   Mild elevations are not infrequent, especially in women. Measure the gamma-GT (GGT) to see if it is of liver or bone origin, (the GGT should be normal) and the calcium and phosphate to exclude osteomalacia. Paget's disease of bone is a common cause of elevation but it can be confined to one bone and difficult to locate

Urea   3.0–8.8 mmol/l
The normal range should be regarded as unchanged in old age, but many older people have renal impairment; see comments under glomerular filtration rate (GFR)

Creatinine   (in µmol/l) <1.5 × body wt (kg)
The normal range depends on body mass and is complex. The above is a quick rule of thumb. The absolute level of serum creatinine (or its reciprocal) is adequate for monitoring changes in GFR. For measurement of GFR, do a short creatinine clearance or use the formula:

$$GFR = \frac{(140 - age) \times body\ wt\ (kg)}{plasma\ creatinine\ (\mu mol)}$$

T4   70–140 nmol/l
hormones   There may be significant variations in the level of thyroid-binding-globulin (TBG) in old age. When clinical and biochemical measures of thyroid function do not seem to agree, either measure TBG, or free hormone levels, or measure TSH as an arbiter. The 'sick euthyroid syndrome' is very common in the acutely ill elderly. The drug amiodarone is commonly used in old age and has complex effects on thyroid function

Digoxin   1.0–2.0 nmol/l
Toxicity may occur with a total level in the accepted therapeutic range for younger subjects

Electrocardiograph (ECG)
Some reduction in QRS voltage, i.e. the criteria for LVH should be relaxed compared with younger subjects, absolute criteria not known

Chest radiograph
No change to the measurements in younger ages (i.e. an enlarged heart implies heart disease)

CHAPTER 4

The presentation and management of mental disease in older people

Catherine Oppenheimer

The common mental disorders of old age – the dementing illnesses, depression, anxiety and paranoid states – are covered briefly in this chapter. The emphasis is on dementia, because of the heavy burden it causes for patients, families, the primary care team and social services; and because we now understand much better the pattern of services that it requires.

Assessment

Assessment is a broader concept than diagnosis: it includes an understanding of the patient's life history, personality, and close relationships. These colour the presentation of the illness, influence the choice of treatment, and determine what interventions will be accepted.

In psychiatric assessment, information from the patient is combined with accounts from other sources. Psychiatric illness is apt to distort a patient's own account: through poor memory, despair, elation, lack of insight or confabulation. These distortions in themselves give useful diagnostic clues, provided that the correct facts are known from elsewhere. Without objective information, for example, the depressed patient's fears

of financial disaster may be taken at face value, and an illness be mistaken for a social problem.

The other reason why the views of informants are important is that their perception may actually be part of the problem. An overburdened carer will give an account coloured by their own feelings, and these need equal attention when a management plan is made.

The information given by carers should never be discounted. Early signs of serious psychiatric illness are often detected first by those who know the patient best, and if the doctor cannot find anything wrong at that time, it is wise to reserve judgement and reassess after a few months.

Key points

Psychiatric assessment encompasses:

- information from others
- the patient's subjective account
- observation of mental state signs revealed in the account
- the patient's answers to specific questions concerning their mental state

Diagnosis

Psychiatric diagnosis is founded on a systematic search for evidence in support of diagnostic hypotheses. No one would examine an abdomen simply by stroking it; neither can a mental state be assessed by social conversation. The signs of mental illness must consciously be listened for, and the appropriate questions asked. Without this determined awareness, depression and dementia are easily missed.

Some changes of emphasis are helpful when using the standard psychiatric examination with older people. Ask the patient to tell you briefly the story of his or her life: careful listening will reveal important clues to cognition, mood and insight. You will need some simple framework to remind you to assess relevant aspects of the mental state; this should include the patient's appearance, behaviour, speech, thoughts, mood, perceptions and insight. If there are any doubts about the patient's cognitive abilities (including orientation, language, memory and reasoning), questions specific to these areas should be asked.

There are some useful rules of thumb: for example, patients who complain of poor memory or concentration are often depressed rather than demented, while difficulty in word-finding raises the suspicion of early Alzheimer's disease.

A careful psychiatric assessment takes time, but your efforts will be rewarded by the solid foundation it creates for the future relationship between the patient and yourself.

Standard questionnaires for partial assessments of the mental state have been developed, such as the Mini-Mental State Examination (MMSE) for cognitive assessment, and the Geriatric Depression Scale (GDS) (see Boxes 4.1 and 4.2).

Assessment under the Mental Health Act 1983

The general practitioner's (GP's) role in assessing a patient for emergency admission to hospital under the Mental Health Act is much the same whatever the patient's age. The Approved Social Worker is the authority on the proper use of the Act, while a psychiatrist and the patient's GP provide the definitive opinion on the patient's mental state. The three key requirements are as follows.

1 The patient must have a mental illness (or one of the other conditions specified in the Act).

2 There must be a risk to the patient's health or safety or the safety of others.

3 There must be reasons why treatment outside hospital would not be appropriate.

Compulsory admissions under Section 2 or 3 of the Act are most often needed for severe depressions and paranoid states. Dementia is also a mental illness and can justify admission under this Act. In practice, many patients with dementia are admitted informally, though strictly speaking they may not be competent to give real consent to their admission.

In addition, guardianship under Section 7 of the Mental Health Act is a valuable option. It can be a formal safeguard for the care of a demented person living at home, who says she needs no help, while actually accepting the visits of persuasive care staff. Also, under guardianship there is a procedure that can be used to set aside a relative who unreasonably obstructs the provision of help to a patient in need.

Difficult ethical and legal issues surround the care of mentally ill older people, who are vulnerable to neglect and exploitation. Physical, emotional, sexual and financial abuse of older people are increasingly recognized. Detailed knowledge of the Mental Health Act and of local procedures is needed in such cases, and the specialist services should be involved, notably Social Services and Old Age Psychiatry teams.

The dementing illnesses

Definition

The defining features of a dementing illness are a global cognitive impairment (i.e. more than one faculty is impaired), in the absence of impaired consciousness. Where consciousness is impaired, the diagnosis, by definition, is a delirium (also known as acute confusional state).

The diagnostic guidelines of the International Classification of Diseases (ICD 10) give a thumbnail clinical description of these two conditions:

Dementia: '... evidence of a decline in both memory and thinking which is sufficient to

Box 4.1: The 'mini-mental state examination' (MMSE)

Orientation	Score
1 Can you tell me what	
year it is?	1
season?	1
date?	1
day?	1
month?	1

2 Can you tell me where we are?
what town (or village)? — 1
what street (or hospital)? — 1
what house (or ward)? — 1
what county? — 1
what country? — 1

Registration

3 'I would like you to remember three things for me. The three things are... — 3 (name three objects, taking 1 second to say each)'. Then ask the patient all three, after you have said them. Give one point for each correct answer. Then repeat the three objects until the patient can repeat them all. 'Now please keep remembering those three, and I will ask you about them later'.

Attention and calculation

4 Serial sevens. Give one point — 5 for each correct answer. Stop after five answers. Alternative: spell 'WORLD' backwards.

Recall

5 Ask for the names of the three — 3 objects learned in question **3**. Give one point for each correct answer.

Language — Score

6 Point to a pencil and a watch, — 2 say 'Can you tell me what that is called?'

7 Ask the patient to repeat 'No — 1 ifs, ands, or buts'.

8 Ask the patient to follow a — 3 three-stage command: 'Please take this piece of paper in your right hand, fold it in half, and put in on the floor'.

9 Ask the patient to read and — 1 follow the written command: 'CLOSE YOUR EYES'. (Write the command in large clear capitals.)

10 Ask the patient to write a sentence — 1 of his or her choice. (To score correctly, the sentence must contain a subject and a verb. Spelling mistakes do not matter.)

11 Draw the design below and — 1 ask the patient to copy it. (Draw it with sides of 1.5 cm at least. To score correctly, each pentagon must have 5 sides and the intersecting sides must form a quadrangle.)

TOTAL = 30

Cut off point for probable cognitive impairment is 24.

Source: Folstein MF, Folstein SE and McHugh PR (1975) 'Mini-mental state: A practical method for grading the cognitive state of patients for the clinician. *J Psychiatr Res* **12**:189–98.

Box 4.2: Geriatric depression scale (GDS) (short form)

Name _____   Date _____

Choose the best answer for how you have felt over the past week:

1	Are you basically satisfied with your life?	YES / <u>NO</u>
2	Have you dropped many of your activities and interests?	<u>YES</u> / NO
3	Do you feel that your life is empty?	<u>YES</u> / NO
4	Do you often get bored?	<u>YES</u> / NO
5	Are you in good spirits most of the time?	YES / <u>NO</u>
6	Are you afraid that something bad is going to happen to you?	<u>YES</u> / NO
7	Do you feel happy most of the time?	YES / <u>NO</u>
8	Do you often feel helpless?	<u>YES</u> / NO
9	Do you prefer to stay at home, rather than going out and doing new things?	<u>YES</u> / NO
10	Do you feel you have more problems with memory than most?	<u>YES</u> / NO
11	Do you think it is wonderful to be alive now?	YES / <u>NO</u>
12	Do you feel pretty worthless the way you are now?	<u>YES</u> / NO
13	Do you feel full of energy?	YES / <u>NO</u>
14	Do you feel that your situation is hopeless?	<u>YES</u> / NO
15	Do you think that most people are better off than you are?	<u>YES</u> / NO

(Answers indicating depression are underlined. A score of more than five such answers indicates probable depressive illness.)

Yesavage JA, Brink TL, Rose TL and Lum O (1983) Development and validation of a geriatric depression screening scale: a preliminary report. *J Psychiatric Research* **17**:37–49.

impair personal activities of daily living … . The impairment of memory typically affects the registration, storage, and retrieval of new information, but previously learned and familiar material may also be lost, particularly in the later stages… there is also impairment of thinking and of reasoning capacity, and a reduction in the flow of ideas. The processing of incoming information is impaired… it becomes difficult to attend to more than one stimulus at a time, such as taking part in a conversation with several persons, and to shift the focus of attention from one topic to another.

If dementia is the sole diagnosis, evidence of clear consciousness is required. However, a double diagnosis of delirium superimposed on dementia is common.'

Delirium: 'For a definite diagnosis, symptoms, mild or severe, should be present *in each one* of the following areas:

(a) *impairment of consciousness and attention* (… reduced ability to direct, focus, sustain, and shift attention)

(b) *global disturbance of cognition* (perceptual distortion, illusions and hallucinations; impairment of abstract thinking and comprehension…; impairment of immediate recall and of recent memory but with relatively intact remote memory; disorientation for time as well as place and person)

(c)   *psychomotor disturbances* (hypo- or hyper-activity and unpredictable shifts from one to the other; increased reaction time; increased or decreased flow of speech; enhanced startle reaction)

(d)   *disturbance of the sleep–wake cycle* (insomnia or, in severe cases, total sleep loss or reversal of the sleep–wake cycle; daytime drowsiness; nocturnal worsening of symptoms; disturbing dreams or nightmares, which may continue as hallucinations after awakening)

(e)   *emotional disturbances*, e.g. depression, anxiety or fear, irritability, euphoria, apathy, or wondering perplexity.

The onset is usually rapid, the course diurnally fluctuating, and the total duration of the condition less than 6 months.'

Delirium is usually due to physical illness, sometimes in combination with a mild dementia previously unrecognized. But in vascular dementia, and in the dementia of Parkinson's disease, episodes of delirium can occur without any additional physical cause (such as infection of chest or urinary tract) being found.

Presentation

In early dementia, common presentations are:

- ill-defined concerns felt by relatives

- patient's awareness that 'something is wrong'

- forgetfulness, especially for recent events

- deteriorating performance at work

- errors in social behaviour

- post-retirement 'apathy' (sometimes labelled 'depression')

- unexpected emotional responses (e.g. tearfulness, anger).

In Alzheimer's disease and in frontal-lobe dementia, the onset of difficulties is typically gradual, while in vascular dementia the onset can be abrupt, sometimes following a cerebral infarct, sometimes heralded by episodes of confusion.

Though memory loss is a classical feature of dementia, the absence of memory loss does not rule out the diagnosis. In frontal-lobe dementia, and sometimes in early Alzheimer's disease, memory may be spared while signs appear in other cognitive domains:

- language impairment (especially difficulty in word-finding)

- errors in visuo-spatial tasks (such as following a map)

- problems in carrying out relatively complex actions (e.g. changing a plug)

- impairment of higher-order cerebral function (e.g. planning ahead, emotional understanding, judging social situations).

In early frontal-lobe dementia, loss of judgement and of emotional sensitivity may be the only signs of something wrong. The person may not appear ill at all: instead he/she is seen as feckless, disagreeable, stubborn or unfeeling. Major family stresses or trivial illegal acts can ensue. The GP's ability to recognize the illness underlying the social crisis is crucial, so that referral and diagnosis can occur in time to prevent a wholesale breakdown of the patient's social supports.

Alcohol

Alcohol complicates recognition of a dementing illness. Sometimes heavy drinking is itself the cause of the cerebral damage; more often, a dementing illness impairs the control of drinking, so that alcohol toxicity amplifies confusion due to the illness. Both possibilities need to be recognized.

Diagnosis

Any interview with an older patient (not necessarily demented) tests their ability to talk with relevance, coherence, accurate use of detail, and correct choice of words.

However, competence in these areas does not prove that all is well. A patient may in all sincerity give an account of a busy and well-organized life, which is later revealed by informants to be quite untrue. A disastrous decline in their practical abilities has been concealed by the preservation of their verbal skills.

Specific questions and standard tests

A standard test of cognitive ability such as the MMSE is usually well accepted (and often enjoyed) by patients, if they understand that it is part of the doctor's routine practice. The test should be administered with encouragement and humour (without being patronizing), and errors passed over lightly.

The most sensitive test of memory loss is the recall of new information after distraction (e.g. remembering the names of three objects after spelling backwards, as in the MMSE). It involves coding for storage and retrieval: abilities which are affected early and severely in Alzheimer's disease.

Information from others

Subtle changes may be detected by families long before the diagnosis is clear, or the patient realizes there is a problem. Conversely, some carers adapt unconsciously to the gradually increasing needs of a patient, and can be startlingly unaware of quite serious impairment.

Therefore, attend seriously to the information given by carers, but weigh it against your own evaluation, and seek information from other sources where evidence conflicts. Make sure to give carers the opportunity to speak to you in private, or they may conceal facts so as not to upset the patient.

Investigations

Dementia is a clinical syndrome, diagnosed on clinical findings. Investigations help to exclude other diagnoses, may suggest aetiology, and detect other conditions (such as anaemia or hypothyroidism) which add to the patient's disability.

Routine laboratory screening in dementia should include:

- blood count, folic acid and B_{12} estimation
- blood biochemistry, liver and thyroid function
- syphilis serology
- urinalysis.

Further investigations, such as computerized tomography and single photon emission computed tomography (SPECT) scanning, are usually arranged after specialist referral. Very occasionally this will reveal a manageable cause for the 'dementia' such as meningioma.

Referral for specialist opinion

Old-age psychiatry teams welcome early referrals, and most teams accept open referral, through either the community psychiatric nurse or the psychiatrist.

Management

Each patient needs a plan tailored specifically to his or her circumstances. The essence of a good management plan (formally enshrined in the Care Programme Approach) is:

- thorough initial assessment
- regular review to ensure that the plan adapts to changing need
- clarity of the roles of different participants
- one person identified as key worker, with responsibility for coordinating the input of all the others.

At some stage in the illness, the GP and the primary care team, a care manager from social services, and a community psychiatric nurse from the old-age psychiatry service (if not others as well) are likely to be involved in the patient's care; and good teamwork between them is essential.

Management issues that arise commonly include the following.

Breaking the news

The diagnosis is often suspected by carers, and is usually shared with them when it is confirmed. They may ask for the patient not to be told, fearing it will cause needless distress or make the task of caring more difficult. Sometimes the diagnosis comes as a relief rather than a shock: the incomprehensible changes in the patient were more distressing to them than knowing the true explanation.

Giving information, and establishing contact with other agencies

Patients and carers need to be fully briefed about all the different local sources of help. Various ways of relieving the burden on the carer, or of sharing their responsibility, have been invented: these include home care (by visiting care staff), day care, sitting services, night visits, and respite admissions; these may be provided by social services, the health service, independent or voluntary agencies – the exact arrangements differ in different places.

National voluntary organizations, such as the Alzheimer's Disease Society, are important sources of information and support to patients and their carers (see further reading list on p. 64).

Finances

The best way of avoiding later financial complications is for the patient to arrange (preferably through a solicitor) an Enduring Power of Attorney (EPA). This must be drawn up while the patient (the 'donor') is able to understand what the EPA means. When the patient becomes too ill to understand the decisions being made on his behalf, the EPA must be registered with the Court of Protection. Thereafter, the attorney is answerable to the Court.

Many other financial issues may arise, on which the carer will need advice: Age Concern and the Alzheimer's Disease Society can give helpful information, and social services care managers are often necessarily involved.

Driving

Driving in dementia is a difficult issue. Useful guidance is given in the publication *At a Glance Guide to the Current Medical Standards of*

Fitness to Drive, produced by the Driving and Vehicle Licensing Agency, whose medical advisers also give advice over the telephone to doctors (Tel. 01792 783784).

Living arrangements

When difficulties in managing day-to-day life begin, a move to sheltered accommodation or to live with relatives may seem a good solution. Alas, the advantages are often illusory. The doctor can help by ensuring that:

- the patient's abilities and disabilities are clearly established

- the relatives have taken time to consider all foreseeable consequences of a move

- social services have made an independent assessment of the patient's needs and of local resources that could support him or her.

Supporting carers

Surveys of carers have shown that the GP is their most valued source of help and support. Especially in the following ways:

- willingness to be available, to understand, and simply to listen when distress cannot be remedied

- offering time to the carer to discuss problems in private

- attention to the carer's own health (physical and psychological)

- affirmation that the carer is looking after the patient well (often carers worry that others would care better than they do)

- helping with planning ahead

- helping with solving problems

- sharing the burden of responsibility with the carer

- knowing when to say 'enough is enough' (when the carer herself cannot see it).

Understandably, carers do not always readily accept help, or make it easy for others to help them. They may be afraid of upsetting the person they care for, of destabilizing a situation under

Table 4.1: Comparison of drugs used in suspicion and paranoia

	Haloperidol	Thioridazine
Antipsychotic potency	High	Mild
Sedative effect	Low	High
Parkinsonian side-effects	Can be severe	Low risk
Cumulative effect	Yes (beware)	No
Available as liquid	Yes	Yes
Initial (trial) dose	0.5–1 mg	10–25 mg
Likely upper limit	1–2 mg bd	50 mg tds

precarious control, of causing the patient to be 'put away', or of incurring unaffordable expense.

Behavioural problems and medication

Medication has a limited part to play in dementia. Social and nursing measures are usually far more important, but there are three complications that need treatment with drugs: suspicion and paranoia; depression; insomnia.

Suspicion and paranoia

People with delirium or dementia may be very frightened (especially when they have some awareness of the change they are undergoing), and paranoid explanations for their experiences may develop. Reassurance is usually ineffective if the feelings are intense, but medication may be accepted. Thioridazine and haloperidol serve as examples in choosing the most appropriate drug for a given patient (Table 4.1).

Where the prime need is to achieve sedation, thioridazine should be tried first, starting cautiously and titrating the dose against the response. One dose in the early evening (when fear and suspicion tend to be greatest) and another at bedtime may be enough, and avoids over-sedation in the day.

Visual hallucinations

Visual hallucinations can occur in Alzheimer's disease, and are common in the dementia of Parkinson's disease. Treatment with neuroleptics can cause severe side-effects, but sometimes a

cautious reduction in the anti-Parkinsonian medication will work; other medication (such as the newer neuroleptics) is best tried under specialist supervision.

Depression

Depression is hard to detect in dementia. Unhappiness, poor sleep or loss of appetite, agitation and disturbed behaviour can indicate its presence. The best test may be by trial of carefully monitored antidepressant medication. The tricyclic antidepressants cause troublesome side-effects; the SSRI can increase agitation in some (but are well-tolerated by others). Trazodone is useful, being well-tolerated and moderately sedating, but it takes effect over several weeks so any trial should not be prematurely abandoned.

Disturbed sleep

Disturbed sleep in a patient leads to disturbed sleep in the carer, who will not be able to take daytime naps to compensate. A well-structured, happily occupied day will help a patient to sleep better at night, but this may not be achievable. Thioridazine or trazodone can be used for their sedative effects; benzodiazepines are generally avoided at this stage (they can cause confusion and falls).

Behavioural complications

Behavioural complications in dementia include hyperactivity and 'wandering', intractable night-time restlessness, persistent calling and shouting, aggressive behaviour, reclusiveness and refusal of help, and incontinence not manageable by simple nursing measures. Ask for specialist advice with these difficult problems.

The terminal stage in dementia

As dementia progresses, the patient becomes increasingly dependent, and physical difficulties – frailty and immobility – add to this. Apraxia and agnosia can cause distressing problems for carers, and are often misunderstood by them. (It helps to know that the patient urinates in a wastepaper basket because he misperceives it, rather than because he wants to make trouble.) Difficulties increase when the patient construes assistance as an intrusion into his private space, and fiercely resists it. This is hurtful to carers even when they understand it, and makes their task even harder.

Ultimately, the stage is reached when institutional care has to be considered. Family carers often suffer guilt and a sense of failure at this point, however impossible the burden of care at home has become, and they may need the GP or the specialist team to make the final decision for them.

Ideally, the GP's care continues through into the nursing home, where emphasis should be on the maintenance of the best possible quality of life. For example, benzodiazepines may now be useful in relieving generalized anxiety, or the distress of an upsetting event such as an enema, or a bath. Often, other medication can be gradually withdrawn.

Decisions about the use of antibiotics in intercurrent illness, or the use of life-saving interventions, will be made after discussion with close relatives and the nursing staff. Where a decision not to give any curative treatment is made, attention to the relief of symptoms is still essential.

The late phase of dementia can last months, or sometimes years. These months should contain as many enjoyable experiences for the patient as possible: simple things such as a favourite food, familiar music, or visits outside the home.

It is often painful for family members to maintain contact with the patient, when they are not giving direct care, and the patient no longer recognizes them or even reacts to their visits. The staff of the home and the GP can help to bridge this distressing gap by putting effort into good communication with the family, and encouraging their participation in all important decisions, so that they still feel involved in the patient's welfare.

Depression in old age

The word 'depression' can embrace everything from a transient low mood in response to the ordinary stresses of life, to a life-threatening delusional illness.

In the International Classification of Diseases (ICD 10) the diagnostic criteria for depressive disorder begin with the following:

Depressive disorder: 'In typical depressive episodes (mild, moderate or severe) the individual usually suffers from depressed mood, loss of interest and enjoyment, and reduced energy leading to increased fatiguability and diminished activity. Marked tiredness after only slight effort is common. Other common symptoms are:
(a) reduced concentration and attention
(b) reduced self-esteem and self-confidence
(c) ideas of guilt and unworthiness
(d) bleak and pessimistic ideas of the future
(e) ideas or acts of self-harm or suicide
(f) disturbed sleep
(g) diminished appetite.

The lowered mood varies little from day to day, and is often unresponsive to circumstances, yet may show a characteristic diurnal variation as the day goes on… . In some cases, anxiety, distress, and motor agitation may be more prominent at times than the depression, and the mood change may also be masked by added features such as irritability, excess consumption of alcohol, histrionic behaviour, and exacerbation of pre-existing phobic or obsessional symptoms, or by hypochondriacal preoccupations… .'

Depressive symptoms are found in 20% of patients over the age of 65, and depressive disorder (i.e. the full-blown picture of depressive illness) in about 5%. Detecting and treating depression is not always easy, and although detection rates in general practice have increased significantly in the last few decades, detection does not always lead to effective treatment.

Those at highest risk are people who are physically ill, abusing alcohol, bereaved, living alone or in poverty, chronically disabled or in institutional care. All but the last three also have an increased risk of suicide.

Diagnosis of depression

The classical somatic symptoms of depressive illness (disturbed sleep pattern and appetite, weight loss, loss of energy, loss of libido, impaired concentration and memory) are also found in physical illness in old age, so they may not point so directly to the diagnosis as do the psychological signs of depression, and alterations in behaviour and speech.

Anhedonia – the inability to experience pleasure (in things which the patient formerly enjoyed) – is an invaluable sign of depression where physical illness or disability obscure the evaluation of other signs.

Doctors should beware of the patient who has 'every reason to feel depressed' – this is not a reason for avoiding the diagnosis of depressive illness. Untreated depression will only prolong the patient's suffering and undermine the strength they need to resolve their other difficulties.

Differential diagnosis

Depression may be mislabelled in a number of different ways, depending on which are the most prominent symptoms (Table 4.2).

Treatment of depression

Modern treatments for depression are usually effective and well-tolerated, and the cost of missed diagnosis or failure to treat is measured in suicide, avoidable distress, burden on carers and unnecessary dependence.

Both physical treatments (medication and electroconvulsive therapy (ECT)) and psychological treatments (such as cognitive therapy or

Table 4.2: Symptoms and differential diagnosis of depression

Symptom	Differential diagnosis
Weight loss, anorexia	Physical illness
Somatic complaints	Hypochondriasis
Agitation, restlessness	Anxiety state
Intensely demanding behaviour	'Hysterical' personality
Sleep disturbance	Simple insomnia
Impaired concentration	Dementia
Depressive delusions	Paranoid illness
Self-neglect	Freely chosen lifestyle

supportive psychotherapy) are used for depressive illness in old age. The more severe the illness, the more important is initial physical treatment, because the illness itself affects thinking and concentration, on which psychological treatments rely.

There is a wide choice of antidepressants. The classical tricyclics are still as effective as any other medication, but their side-effects (cardiotoxicity, postural hypotension, constipation, dry mouth) are troublesome in old age, and they are dangerous in overdose. Safer drugs include lofepramine, the SSRIs, moclobemide, trazodone and venlafaxine. The therapeutic effect of these drugs is broadly the same, but they differ in their typical side-effects.

If the patient refuses treatment, is experiencing suicidal thoughts or delusions, is neglecting to eat and drink and losing weight, or if treatment is ineffective, then you must refer them for specialist advice. Admission to hospital can offer more support and closer monitoring than can be given outside, and a wider range of treatment options is available – including ECT, which is still the safest and most effective treatment for depression in older people.

Hypomania and manic-depressive illness

Hypomania and mania are certainly seen in older people, but generally only in people with recognized manic-depressive disorder over the course of their lives. Rarely, a physical illness or medication (particularly steroid treatment) can precipitate hypomania. Frontal-lobe dementia can present with a clinical picture resembling mania – with voluble speech, shallow jocularity and socially disinhibited behaviour. It is difficult to supervise treatment of a patient with manic illness in the community, and the specialist services should always be involved.

Anxiety states

Most anxiety among older people is seen in those who have been anxious all their lives. The onset of anxiety in old age can be triggered by a frightening event (such as a burglary), by bereavement – especially the loss of a person on whom the patient depended for reassurance – or by an episode which undermines the person's confidence, such as giddiness resulting in a fall. Lifelong anxiety can be expressed through hypochondriacal fears and preoccupation with physical health, and old age may increase those fears. Anxiety may be the presenting symptom of another illness: commonly depression, but sometimes an early dementia.

Diagnosis of an anxiety state

Making a diagnosis of an anxiety state, and distinguishing between a specific phobia, generalized anxiety, panic attacks, or agoraphobia, depends on establishing:

- the presence of physical symptoms of anxiety (racing heart, breathlessness, sweating, giddiness, dry mouth)

- the presence of anxious thoughts (fear of dying, fainting, having a stroke)

- the relationship between the anxiety and circumstances which precipitate it or relieve it (e.g. agoraphobia is relieved by returning to a safe place or a safe person).

Management of anxiety

Management of anxiety is mainly psychological, although a sedative antidepressant can be useful even when there are no depressive symptoms. Benzodiazepines are better avoided because they readily induce dependence in these circumstances.

Psychological measures include education of the patient about anxiety, so that the physical symptoms can be accepted and not seen as signs of catastrophe; training in the technique of relaxation, including slow breathing techniques for patients who are liable to hyperventilate under stress; encouraging a carefully graduated, step-by-step return to the feared situation, with detailed feedback and praise at each step.

There are many excellent self-help books on anxiety, and patients should be encouraged to consult their local library for these.

Paranoid states

Paranoid thinking is most common in people with a long-established 'prickly' personality, prone to suspiciousness and precarious social relationships. It is also found where there is a history of schizophrenia, and sometimes early in a dementing illness. Lastly, a paranoid illness with pronounced delusional ideas and hallucinations can arise in old age without any obvious predisposing cause.

Paranoid beliefs can lead a patient into disruptive, embarrassing or even dangerous behaviour. Specialist advice is usually needed, and involuntary admission to hospital under the Mental Health Act may be required. Patients are usually distressed by their delusional convictions and by what they perceive as hostile and damaging acts by others, but they will rarely accept that they are ill and need treatment.

There are some useful basic principles in managing a paranoid patient. Let them see that their concerns are being taken seriously and that you respect their account of their beliefs and experiences. You may suggest, gently, that there might be alternative explanations, but do not argue the point. Explain that you believe they may be ill, and listen for any symptoms they acknowledge. They may at least accept that they are exhausted, sleepless or distressed, and if you have secured their trust, they may agree to try medication to relieve such symptoms.

If the patient is willing to accept medication, the choice of anti-psychotic drug will be governed by considerations of potency, freedom from side-effects and safety. Possible choices include thioridazine, trifluoperazine, pimozide and risperidone. The community psychiatric nurse is a valuable support to the GP in managing such patients, backed up by the old-age psychiatric team.

Further reading

Alzheimer's Disease Society (1995) *Dementia in the Community: management strategies for general practice*. Alzheimer's Disease Society, Gordon House, 10 Greencoat Place, London SW1 1PH.

Butler G and Hope T (1995) *Managing your mind: the mental fitness guide*. Oxford University Press, Oxford.

Davis R and Davis B (1989) *My journey into Alzheimer's disease: helpful insights for family and friends*. British edn (1993) published by Scripture Press Foundation (UK) Ltd, Raans Road, Amersham-on-the-Hill, Bucks HP6 6JQ.

Jacoby R and Oppenheimer C (eds) (1997) *Psychiatry in the Elderly*, 2nd edn. Oxford University Press, Oxford.

Mace NL, Rabins PV and Castleton BA (1985) *The thirty-six hour day*. Hodder and Stoughton, with Age Concern, London.

Rachman S and de Silva P (1996) *Panic Disorder: the facts*. Oxford University Press, Oxford.

Wilcock G (1990) *Living with Alzheimer's disease and similar conditions*. Penguin, London.

CHAPTER 5

Prescribing and the older patient in the community

Michael Denham

An eminent Professor of geriatric medicine once said that his greatest therapeutic triumphs were achieved by stopping drugs given by other doctors. There is much to be learnt from this statement. First, the pharmaceutical revolution, which started some 50 years ago, has produced many drugs which can be of great benefit and value to older people provided they are used sensibly. Furthermore, the range of drugs available over the counter (OTC) has changed dramatically in recent years to include many new classes of drugs, such as NSAIDs and H$_2$ antagonists.

Second, there is extensive polypharmacy in older age groups, particularly those living in private residential or nursing homes, whose number has increased steadily in the last 10 to 20 years. In the latter situation, the community pharmacist can have a major role in promoting sensible and safe prescribing.

Third, the statement implies that the reason for stopping drugs is an adverse drug reaction. It is now well recognized that such reactions increase with age. The therapeutic challenge facing all doctors, therefore, is to prescribe sensibly and effectively, steer a course between under- and over-treatment, balance risk and benefit, and above all, avoid causing harm to the patient.

Prescribing patterns for older people

Although elderly people comprise only 18% of the population, they not only receive a disproportionate amount of prescribed medication, but that proportion is increasing. Thus, in 1985 39% of all prescriptions were dispensed to them, compared with 45% in 1995. The number of prescription items per head for older people increased from 14.6 to 21.8 over the same period.[1] There was above-average growth in several therapeutic categories such as cardiovascular, musculoskeletal and gastrointestinal medications, where high proportions of prescriptions were for older people. Much of this prescribing was for repeat medication rather than first prescriptions.

This growth in prescribing for older people makes a significant contribution to the cost of prescribing in primary care. The Family Health Service drugs bill rose from £1130 million in 1983/84 to £2951 million in 1993/94 (a rise of 161% in cash terms; 55% in real terms). Almost half (43%) of this increase over ten years is accounted for by the cost of prescriptions for older people.[1] Changes in demography account for only a small part of the increase. The main factor is an increase in the number of items prescribed per person. The cost of prescribing for older people is therefore not only rising but it is also taking an increasing proportion of drug costs.

Adverse drug reactions

Adverse drug reactions (ADR) remain a very important cause of morbidity in the elderly – a survey by Williamson and Chopin showed that one in ten of all admissions to acute geriatric units were wholly or partly due to drug side-effects.[2] Subsequent studies have reported similar findings.

The total number of ADR yellow-card reports received by the Committee of Safety of Medicines shows an increase with age, particularly when the number of serious ADR reports is expressed per million of first prescriptions received. However, these reports may be an under-representation of the size of the problem, since some adverse drug reactions may be attributed to old age or to disease(s) from which the patient suffers.

There are seven main causes of adverse drug reactions:

1 inadequate clinical assessment

2 inadequate long-term review

3 polypharmacy

4 poor compliance

5 altered pharmacokinetics with age

6 altered pharmacodynamics with age

7 previous adverse reactions.

Inadequate clinical assessment

A major problem facing the general practitioner (GP) can be lack of time. The older person may suffer from many different disabilities or conditions which produce a range of symptoms. This, combined with the non-specific presentation of disease in older people, and sometimes with difficulties in obtaining an accurate history, means that time is required to sort out exactly what is going on. Unfortunately, of course, the doctor is generally under pressure and may be tempted to treat the symptom rather than the disease itself – hence inappropriate medication may be prescribed, e.g. prochlorperazine for

dizziness in the older person is a classic example. Unfortunately, this symptom has many causes, of which middle-ear disease is an unlikely cause in the older person.

Long-term medication

Drugs prescribed for an acute condition may no longer be required once it has resolved. Studies have shown that about a third of drugs given to older people admitted to hospital can be stopped without detriment to the patient either because they were unnecessary or were contraindicated. Audit schemes to improve supervision of long-term medication, therefore, have much to recommend them.

Polypharmacy and inappropriate prescribing

In spite of the difficulties it causes for patients, the problems of compliance and the danger of drug interaction(s) with side-effects, polypharmacy remains widespread. This generally occurs because an elderly person can have many clinical problems and because of failure to clarify the aims of treatment. Elderly people admitted to hospital can be taking as many as 12 different medications, many of which are repeat prescriptions. Studies have shown that approximately 10% of all medications to older persons are contraindicated in relation to the clinical diagnosis or results of clinical tests, e.g. potassium-sparing diuretics in the presence of renal failure.[3]

Poor compliance

Compliance with prescribed medication can present problems for patients – as many as three-quarters of older people make errors in taking their medicine, a quarter of which may be serious.[4] The causes are multiple and frequently inter-linked.

• The patient may make a positive decision not to take the medicine because: the symptoms may have cleared, there may be a lack of improvement, development of side-effects or even lack of faith in the doctor. Alternatively, the patient may be unable to take the medicines because of inability to open the container, read the instructions or confusion about when and how the medicines are to be taken.

- The doctor may be partly to blame because of failure to explain adequately to the patient the need for the medicines and how and when they should be taken, failure to check that the patient can open the container, or through failure to give the correct instructions to the pharmacist, perhaps coupled with a failure to check previous medication the patient has been taking.

- The pharmacist can have problems if the doctor does not give adequate instructions, e.g. indicate how and when the drug is to be taken, resulting in the instruction 'to be taken when directed' being written on the container. The pharmacist also may not be given special instructions to write labels in large print or supply a container which is easy for the patient to open. Unless suitable instructions are given, a child-resistant container will be supplied, which may be impossible for the patient to open.

Since poor compliance can have detrimental effects on the patient, it is essential to try to improve it as follows:

- ensure the patient understands the instructions – both oral and written

- keep the regimen simple

- use as few drugs as possible

- consider use of medication aids, e.g. Dosett box

- ensure regular review of long-term medication

- when in doubt, don't prescribe.

Compliance can be assessed reasonably simply by either direct or indirect methods. Direct methods include measuring blood or urine concentrations of the drug, or metabolite. Unfortunately, this technique is limited to a few drugs such as digoxin, anti-epileptics and some antibiotics, and the value of the results is limited by the rate at which drugs are metabolized, or excreted. The indirect method involves making tablet counts, discussing problems with the patient, assessing demand for new medication or the response to treatment. Although these techniques are not entirely reliable, they present the simplest and most practical way of assessing compliance.

Altered pharmacokinetics and pharmacodynamics

Pharmacokinetics (what the body does to the drug) changes with increasing age. Drug absorption from the gut is more or less unaltered but distribution of the drug within the body can change due to an increase in body fat and reduced lean-body mass seen in old age. The result is that the potential depot for fat-soluble drugs is increased and therefore the half-life lengthened. Many drugs are carried by albumin, the concentration of which often decreases with age, and therefore the total amount of bound drug is reduced. However in the 'steady-state' situation the therapeutic effect of the drug is usually little changed.

The main changes in pharmacokinetics relate to renal and liver function. Glomerular filtration rate deteriorates with age, which means that drugs dependent on the kidney for excretion (such as digoxin) may accumulate if normal adult doses are given. These changes are of particular relevance to drugs with a narrow therapeutic range.

Changes in pharmacodynamics (what the drug does to the body) have been less well studied but it is clear that there is, for example, increasing sensitivity of the brain to drugs which act directly upon it e.g. anaesthetic agents, sedatives, hypnotics, tranquillizers, anti-Parkinsonian agents and antidepressants.

All these changes strongly support the view that the dose of drugs to be given to an elderly person should be carefully titrated to produce the desired therapeutic effect. If in doubt, start with a low dose and increase slowly.

Previous adverse drug reactions

It is important, as part of any drug history, to enquire about any previous drug reactions. Such data need to be inserted in the patient's records and considered whenever new medications are to be prescribed. Failure to note such information can lead to unfortunate results.

Over-the-counter medication and its relevance to prescribing

Over-the-counter (OTC) medication has been available for many years. Many adults use these drugs to treat common illnesses and, therefore, they will develop increasing importance in the future as the flow of new and more powerful medicines (usually in lower doses than when prescribed) are converted from prescriber-only medicines (POM) to pharmacy (P) medicines. This process began to increase in importance in the early 1990s when the non-steroidal anti-inflammatory drugs, such as ibuprofen, and cimetidine, an H_2 antagonist, became available over the counter.

Currently, about £1 billion is spent in the UK on OTC medication. Most of this is spent on respiratory medicines, laxatives and antacids. Studies in the UK suggest that, in general, the use of OTC drugs increases with age and that more women than men take such medicine.

The reasons patients give for taking these medications are multifactorial and include the fact that the OTC medicine may be cheaper than the NHS prescription, is not available on a prescription, and is convenient. Unwillingness to disturb the doctor because the illness is not severe enough, or the medicine has been used successfully before are also reasons.

So far, there are no reported serious adverse drug reactions or interactions attributed to OTC medicines but it should be remembered that three-quarters of patients do not discuss OTC medication with their GP so the potential for adverse drug reactions, interactions and confusion is considerable. Furthermore, a quarter of patients who take OTC medicines to treat an illness are already taking prescribed medicines for the same illness from their doctor.

Community pharmacist

The community pharmacist has a major role in advising patients about health problems, reinforcing advice from the doctor, as well as providing a dispensing service. It is perhaps not well recognized just how substantial an advisory role the community pharmacist has. Approximately 6 million people visit a pharmacist in the UK each day and about 1 million of these visits involve medication enquiries.

Some community pharmacists have developed a close working relationship with managers of independent homes giving advice on drug safety, providing dispensing systems such as Nomad or Manrex and improving staff knowledge about drugs and medication control.

Community pharmacists are frequently involved in Disposal of Unwanted Medicine and Poison (DUMP) campaigns. The success of these campaigns in identifying large quantities of unwanted medicines does tend to suggest major problems of compliance and inappropriate or unnecessary prescribing by the doctor.

Nurse prescribing

Currently, certain groups of nurses such as health visitors, community nurses and diabetic nurses can prescribe from a small range of drugs, as well as certain items of equipment or appliances. The specialist knowledge such nurses possess does allow them to advise GPs in specific areas of patient care. In the future, this role will enlarge following the passage of the Prescription of Medical Products by Nurses Act in 1992, with the setting up of subsequent pilot studies to examine a possible expanded prescribing role.

Prescribing for the continuing-care patient

With well over half a million elderly people in continuing care, the workload of medical care being placed on the GP is steadily increasing, particularly those working in retirement areas, where some general practices may have patients in ten or more nursing homes.

Polypharmacy in nursing homes is widespread, with four out of every five patients on medications and with many patients being prescribed a mean of three to four medicines.[5,6] The potential for adverse drug reactions, drug/drug interactions and inappropriate medications is considerable. Unfortunately, the use of sedation remains widespread – nearly two-thirds of patients in one study of nursing homes were prescribed psychotropic drugs. The situation to avoid is that found in the USA, where sedation is used to 'switch the patient out with the light'. Many studies have shown that large numbers of residents of homes are prescribed potentially interacting drug combinations, in particular drugs with addictive sedative or anticholinergic effects. All these problems may be compounded by less than satisfactory dispensing arrangements in some nursing homes which have been identified by the United Kingdom Central Council for Nursing,

Midwifery and Health Visiting (UKCC). Studies have also shown that prescribing patterns between nursing homes with similar types of patients can vary widely, suggesting differing patterns of prescribing by individual doctors.

While the responsibilities for prescribing and dispensing of drugs are quite clear, the responsibilities for administration of drugs have been the subject of debate. In residential homes the unqualified staff have no defined roles or responsibilities and manage medication according to the requirements of the Registered Homes Act, 1984. Difficulties can arise when patients are self-medicating. In nursing homes, the nursing staff are responsible for the administration of medication according to the standards set by the UKCC.

Registration authorities often employ pharmacists to visit nursing homes to check on the handling of drugs but, unfortunately, there are as yet no agreed national standards. The situation in residential homes may be less than satisfactory since some social service departments have been unable to carry out the statutory number of visits due to lack of trained or adequate staff and even now some departments have yet to draw up their own standard systems.

The role of the doctor in long-stay homes is complex. He should maintain good communications with the care staff. He should be involved in assessment and monitoring of the clinical state of his patients, and prescribing as appropriate, supported by periodic audit. Quality of medical care may be helped if only one or two doctors look after a home rather than many since this should allow agreement between them and the head of the home on standards and policies relating, for example, to the management of incontinence or the treatment of pressure sores. As always, good records are vital for clinical and medico-legal reasons.

Conclusion

Sensible prescribing

There are many factors which influence doctors in their prescribing habits – these include the attitude of the patient and/or the carer, as well as the doctors' knowledge base and experience, and any other external influences placed on them. Patients and/or their carers may have their

own expectations of how they should be treated. Their own beliefs may influence what they expect. Their culture and previous medical treatment may further alter expectations. The doctor will be influenced by their own previous experience and training in the management of a particular condition, and each will probably have a personal or practice formulary from which to prescribe. External influences on the doctor include postgraduate education, local formularies, practice audit of drug prescribing, peer-group pressure, input from independent medical/pharmacological officers of the health authorities and visits from drug representatives. Much, however, depends on a good level of communication between the doctor and their patients.

The pattern of doctor prescribing within primary care is also likely to be influenced by a range of external audit measures now available. Until recently, a GP was able to prescribe without budgetary limitations. However, in the past few years there have been major changes. Fundholding practices now have direct purchasing powers and have a prescribing budget calculated by the independent purchasing authority. Fundholders are encouraged to develop their own formularies which may be constructed with the help of the independent medical and pharmaceutical advisers employed by the FHSA. General practitioners are now also provided with PACT data which list the practice's prescribing patterns for drugs, dressings and appliances. The application of the audit cycle to prescribing patterns may enable the practice to produce savings which can be transferred to other aspects of patient care.

References

1 Department of Health (1995) Data from Statistical Department.
2 Williamson J and Chopin JM (1980) Adverse reactions to prescribed drugs in the elderly: a multicentre investigation. *Age Ageing* **9**:73–80.
3 Gosney M, Vellodi C, Tallis R et al. (1989) Inappropriate prescribing in part II Residential Homes. *Health Trends* **21**:129–30.
4 Schwartz D, Wane M, Zeitz L et al. (1962) Medication errors made by elderly chronically ill patients. *American J Public Health* **52**: 2018–29.

Key points

Prescribing for the older person is not always straightforward and frequently considerable care is required. The rules are:

- make an accurate diagnosis

- assess the pharmacokinetics and pharmacodynamics of the drug in relation to the particular patient

- keep the drug regimen simple, using as few drugs as possible

- make sure the patient understands when and how to take the medication

- consider the use of medication aids

- review the patient's medication regularly

- maintain a personal or practice formulary

- audit personal or practice patterns of prescribing regularly

- when in doubt, don't prescribe

5 Nolan L and O'Malley K (1989) The need for a more rational approach to drug prescribing for elderly people in nursing homes. *Age Ageing* **18**:52–60.

6 Weedle PB, Postan JW and Parish PA (1990) Drug prescribing in residential homes for elderly people in the United Kingdom. *DICP The Annals of Pharmacotherapy* **24**:553–6.

Further reading

An extensive review of medication in older people is to be found in the Royal College of Physician's report on *Medication for Older People* (1997).

CHAPTER 6

Nutrition of older people

Helen Molyneux

'Good nutrition contributes to the health of elderly people and to their ability to recover from illness'.[1] It is projected that the number of people over pensionable age will exceed 16 million by the year 2031, more than double the number in 1961.[2] Focus on nutrition is becoming increasingly important. Ultimately this may lessen the burden of health care costs by enabling elderly people to remain independent as long as possible and overall improving their quality of life.[3]

Nutritionally, it is important to consider elderly people according to biological and not chronological age. As their dependence increases, so the nutritional status of elderly people in the UK declines.[4] It is important to consider each elderly person on an individual basis to ensure their nutrition is optimized.

Factors affecting nutritional status in elderly people can be broadly categorized into three areas:

1 intrinsic factors

2 pathological factors

3 extrinsic factors.

This chapter reviews how these factors may affect the nutrition of elderly people and suggests practical ways to help recognize and address dietary problems.

Intrinsic factors

Intrinsic factors can be defined as the naturally occurring ageing processes which may affect nutritional status.

Composition of the body

Several changes occur within the body with increasing age. Lean-body mass and total body water decrease, whilst total body fat increases. This change in the body's composition leads to a decrease in basal metabolic rate (BMR) which translates into a lower requirement for energy from food. However, the requirement for other nutrients remains consistent with those in younger adults.[5]

Renal function

With ageing there is a decreased blood flow to the kidneys and a decreased glomerular filtration rate. A decrease in anti-diuretic hormone (ADH) sensitivity results in the kidneys being unable to conserve sodium and water as effectively as the younger adult,[6] resulting in less fluid in the body, commonly exacerbated by insufficient fluid intake.

Gastrointestinal system

Taste and smell

With ageing there is a reduction in the ability to taste and smell,[7] often resulting in a diminished food intake.

Mouth

50% of those over 65 years are edentulous.[7] The increase in poor dental health with ageing results in more people using dentures. This in turn may lead to reduced enjoyment and intake of food.

Stomach

Secretion of hydrochloric acid which assists iron absorption diminishes with age.[6] A reduction in the production of intrinsic factor essential for the absorption of vitamin B_{12} also occurs.

Colon

Diminished intestinal blood flow, reduced colonic transport, diminished fluid levels in the body in conjunction with decreased fluid intake often result in constipation.[3] This in turn causes a reduction in appetite and therefore has a negative effect on nutritional status.

Endocrine system

Many endocrine systems undergo functional changes with age, for example, glucose tolerance and satiety, the latter having a direct effect on food intake.

Recommended nutritional intake

In 1991, the Department of Health (DoH) published the dietary reference values (DRV) from the Committee on Medical Aspects of Food Policy (COMA).[8] This provided comprehensive information on the requirements of nutrients for healthy adults. In 1992, the findings of a COMA working party specifically set up to look at the nutritional requirements of healthy elderly people was published,[1] replacing the 1970 COMA report on elderly people.[9] The 1992 report recommended that the DRVs published in the 1991 report on healthy adults[8] be endorsed for elderly people. No information is currently available for the nutritional requirements in acute or chronic illness. Table 6.1 contains the nutritional intakes recommended by the report. To help understand the recommendations, the terms used within the report are quoted below.

- **Lowest reference nutrient intake (LRNI)** – Lowest reference nutrient intake for protein, or

a vitamin, or a mineral. An amount of the nutrient that is enough for only a few people in a group who have low needs.

- **Estimated average requirement (EAR)** – Estimated average requirement of a group of people for energy, or protein, or a vitamin, or mineral. About half will usually need more than the EAR, and half less.

- **Reference nutrient intake (RNI)** – Reference nutrient intake for protein, or a vitamin, or a mineral. An amount of the nutrient that is enough, or more than enough, for about 97% of people in a group. If the average intake of a group is at RNI, then the risk of deficiency in the group is very small.[8]

Pathological factors

Many disease states may indirectly or directly affect nutritional status.

Musculoskeletal disorders

Disorders such as arthritis can lead to inability to prepare food resulting in an intake of limited nutritional content.

Infections

Any infection will result in an increase in BMR, leading to increased energy requirements. However, illness will frequently result in decreased nutritional intake.

Hyperthyroidism and hypothyroidism

Hyperthyroidism raises the BMR, resulting in an increase in energy requirements. Hypothyroidism may reduce BMR and energy requirements.

Wound healing

Successful wound healing can be achieved by the presence of adequate nutritional stores provided by a balanced diet.[10] Many nutrients are essential in the key steps of the wound-healing process, inadequate stores prevent and delay effective wound healing.

Table 6.1: Dietary reference values for the elderly

Nutrient	Sex	Age	Dietary reference value/day
Energy (EAR)	M	60–64	9.93 MJ, 2380 kcal
		65–74	9.71 MJ, 2330 kcal
		75+	8.77 MJ, 2100 kcal
	F	60–64	7.99 MJ, 1900 kcal
			7.96 MJ, 1900 kcal
			7.61 MJ, 1810 kcal
Protein (RNI)	M	50+	53.3 g
	F	50+	46.5 g
Fat	M + F	All	35% of total food energy
Carbohydrate	M + F	All	50% of total food energy dividing into:
			39% starch and intrinsic and milk sugars
			11% non-milk extrinsic sugars
Fibre (DRV)	M + F	All	18 g
Vitamin A			
Retinol equivalents	M	50+	700 µg
(RNI)	F	50+	600 µg
Thiamin (RNI)	M	50+	0.9 mg
	F	50+	0.8 mg
Riboflavin (RNI)	M	50+	1.3 mg
	F	50+	1.1 mg
Niacin (RNI)	M	50+	16 mg
	F	50+	12 mg
Folate (RNI)	M + F	50+	200 µg
Vitamin C (RNI)	M + F	50+	40 mg
Vitamin D (RNI)	M + F	65+	10 µg (from diet or supplements)
Iron (RNI)	M + F	50+	8.7 mg
Calcium (RNI)	M + F	50+	700 mg
Sodium (RNI)	M + F	50+	1600 mg
Potassium (RNI)	M + F	50+	350 mg
Fluid	M + F	All	Minimum 8 cups per day – 1.5 l fluid

Key: M = male, F = female, MJ = megajoules (1 MJ = 239 kcal), kcal = kilocalories (1 kcal = 1 calorie), g = gram, mg = milligrams

Dementia

The severity of the dementia increases the challenge of successfully managing any nutritional consequences.[11] Dementia may also eventually lead to neurogenic dysphagia,[12] and unless carefully monitored may result in rapid weight loss through diminished food intake.

Many other medical conditions may affect nutritional status, many causing anorexia and altered dietary intake.

Extrinsic factors

There are many extrinsic factors that can affect nutritional status. The most common are discussed below.

Drugs

Drugs may affect appetite, gastrointestinal function and interact with foods, known as drug–nutrient interactions. For example, drugs with a high anti-cholinergic effect, such as the tricyclic antidepressants, can produce drug-induced constipation. Long-term anticonvulsant therapy, for example phenytoin or Phenobarbitone, increases the need for folic acid which is found in eggs, green vegetables and oranges. Biguanides, such as metformin decrease the absorption of vitamin B_{12}.

Careful consideration should be given prior to prescribing a drug and devising drug regimens. *Food and medication interactions*[13] is a useful resource for checking drug–nutrient interactions.

Therapeutic diets

Over-restrictive therapeutic diets may contribute to poor nutritional status by reducing the palatability of,[14] for example, modified consistency diets.

Alcohol

Alcohol often takes the place of food in those suffering from alcoholism, resulting in deficiency of many nutrients, e.g. thiamine.[7] Conversely, small amounts of alcohol provided before a meal can stimulate the appetite and enhance nutritional intake.

Dependency

Extensive research has looked at the differences of the nutritional status of institutionalized and house-bound elderly people and those free-living.[12,15,16]

Social isolation

Many elderly people live alone and may have suffered bereavement, the psychological effects of which often result in diminished food intake. Social isolation is independent of financial situation, and affects both poor and rich alike.

Facilities

Other factors affecting the nutritional intake of elderly people are the lack of facilities often due to poverty. Many elderly people may not be able to prepare, or store, food through lack of equipment or space. The lack of facilities can lead to a reduction in the variation of the food consumed and ultimately result in poor nutritional intake.

Environment

Poor environmental conditions, either in the home or nursing home, can reduce appetite. This may be through sights or smells occurring whilst food is being consumed.

The nutritional status of the elderly can be seen to be a constellation of the intrinsic, pathological and extrinsic factors. By improving one factor there may be an indirect positive effect on several other factors and so nutritional status can be improved.

Recognition of elderly at risk of poor nutritional status

It is important to be aware of the factors affecting nutritional status. It is even more important to be able to recognize these factors in elderly people.

The state registered dietitian with an expert knowledge in nutrition and nutritional assessment is the ideal person to assess a person's nutritional needs on an individual basis. Dietitians have unique skills to assess and identify nutritional problems.[17] However, the Community Dietetics Service, as a potential provider of information is under-developed.[18] Educating the multidisciplinary team involved with elderly people to make the appropriate observations could ensure that all people involved with their care (including relatives, friends and neighbours) would quickly be able to identify warning signals that may affect nutritional status. Hence they could create a quicker response for referrals or other actions. Dr Louise Davies has developed a grid system to help in the recognition of elderly people at risk of poor nutritional intake (Figure 6.1).[19]

The grid shows the interrelations between warning signals and risk factors. It enables the assessor to establish and mark with a circle, the most prominent areas of concern for each individual. For example 'living alone' is an acknowledged nutritional risk factor, but that does not mean that all who live alone are malnourished. However, older people who live alone and show signs of any warning signals marked with a dot in the 'living alone' column (e.g. observed depression, missed meals, insufficient food stores) are more likely to be malnourished. If the person is also house-bound or has any other risk factors, the appropriate dots in those columns also need to be circled and there may be good reason to undertake a more detailed assessment so that appropriate action can be implemented swiftly.[19]

Relevant risk factors and observed warning signals

NAME _____

ADDRESS _____

_____

_____

DATE _____

WARNING SIGNALS	living alone	housebound	no regular cooked meals	low mental test score	clinical diagnosis of depression	chronic bronchitis/emphysema	gastrectomy	poor dentition and/or difficulty in swallowing
Recent unintended weight change + or − 3 kg (7 lb)	●	●	●	●	●	●	●	●
Physical disability affecting food shopping, preparation or intake	●	●	●		●	●		
Lack of sunlight		●			●			
Bereavement and/or observed depression/loneliness	●	●	●	●	●	●		
Mental confusion affecting eating	●		●	●				
High alcohol consumption	●		●		●			
Polypharmacy/long-term medication	●		●	●	●			
Missed meals/snacks/fluids	●	●	●	●	●	●	●	●
Food wastage/rejection	●	●	●	●	●	●	●	●
Insufficient food stores at home	●	●	●	●	●	●		
Lack of fruit/juices/vegetables	●	●	●					●
Low budget for food	●		●					
Poor nutritional knowledge		●	●	●			●	●

RISK FACTORS

Reprinted with kind permission of Dr L Davies and The Caroline Walker Trust.[20]

Figure 6.1 Assessment grid

Table 6.2: Ways to improve nutritional intake

Problem	Considerations
Drugs	• Ensure there are no drug–nutrient interactions • Any drugs should be administered at an appropriate time to minimize any side-effects which may prevent adequate nutrient intake e.g. nausea
Therapeutic diets	• Expert advice should be sought from a state registered dietitian to ensure the therapeutic diet is appropriate

Social isolation	• Improving socialization will improve nutritional intake
	• Many options are available, differing in each area, e.g.
	  – luncheon clubs
	  – day centres
	  – 'buddies'

Facilities and knowledge	• Often it is difficult to enhance facilities. However, by maximizing what is available, nutritional intake can be improved, e.g. showing how a microwave works
	• Cookery classes for those with minimal knowledge
	• Meals on wheels
	• Fresh food delivered on a daily basis, e.g. by milkman
	• Store cupboard – the elderly should be encouraged to keep a variety of non-perishable foods in case of illness
	  – milk and milk products (dried milk, long-life milk, milk puddings)
	  – protein-rich foods (tinned meat, fish, pulses)
	  – fruit and vegetables (tinned vegetables)
	  – starchy foods (pasta, instant mash)
	  – extras (e.g. tinned soups)

Environment	• Separate dining area from sleeping and washing areas

Ways to improve nutritional intake

Once the individual has been assessed, it is important to act on the findings. Interventions are aimed at reducing or alleviating risk factors for inadequate nutrition.[21] Table 6.2 describes simple ways in which to improve many of the factors implicated in affecting nutritional status and suggests how to reduce or alleviate them.

It is important to consider each problem in relation to the individual. For example, providing cookery classes will enhance socialization and improve nutritional intake. One means of ensuring elderly people are aware of their nutritional needs and how the ageing process may affect their nutritional status is to target the pre-retirement age group. Many companies now provide nutrition lectures for their employees to help them make appropriate choices through their retirement. This should be made available to all.

Case presentation

The following is a case study to help illustrate what has been discussed throughout this chapter.

Doris is a 73-year-old lady who lives alone in a second-floor flat. She has raised blood pressure and mild heart failure for which her GP has prescribed frumil. Doris passes water several times in the morning and at least twice a night. She is aware that the more she drinks after lunch the more she will get up at night, therefore she only has one cup of tea after lunch. She opens her bowels on average approximately once a week for which she prescribes herself liquid paraffin.

Nutritionally, Doris has one meal a day, in the evening. For this meal she peels the vegetables as she is concerned 'where they have been'. She carries out this preparation first thing in the morning. For breakfast, she eats very little – usually only toast and she has only a small bowl of packet-soup for lunch.

Over the last week she has become increasingly confused, particularly in the evenings and she has had several falls. Doris was admitted to her local district general hospital care for the elderly team. On admission, she was found to be dehydrated and faecally impacted.

Discussion

Doris has many of the factors associated with nutritional risk:

- she lives alone, and has only one meal a day

- her food is low in fibre and other nutrients are lost due to early preparation

- she drinks minimal fluid, to prevent her having to get up in the night

- the decreased sensitivity to ADH with ageing results in increased water being passed, and dehydration

- frumil, a potassium-sparing diuretic. As she has decreased her fluid intake her serum potassium may be rising, contributing to her confusion

- combination of decreased fibre and fluid results in constipation and confusion

- liquid paraffin she self-prescribes may adsorb minerals and therefore may enhance deficiency states.

Treatment

- Clear constipation.
- Increase fibre in her diet.
- Increase fluid.
- Change diuretic.

Together will reduce her confusion and prevent falls.

- Stop liquid paraffin.

- Provide advice on: healthy eating with the DRV guidelines (see Table 6.1).

- Suggest suitable foods for her store cupboard.

- Provide help with her shopping.

- Provide advice regarding food preparation.

- Suggest a luncheon club.

Theoretically, by making these simple changes, Doris's nutritional status can be improved.

However, in practice, it may be more difficult to improve the situation. Doris may be resistant to change or help. It is therefore important to persevere and provide support through change.

Summary

In summary, nutrition is of great importance in elderly people to help each individual remain healthy and independent for longer. Nutritional status is affected by numerous intrinsic, pathological and extrinsic factors. The recognition of these is of vital importance, with a recommended holistic approach being used to enhance nutritional health in elderly people.

References

1 Department of Health (1992) *The Nutrition of Elderly People. Report on Health and Social Subjects No. 43.* Report of the Working Group on the Nutrition of Elderly People of the Committee on Medical Aspects of Food Policy. HMSO, London.

2 Central Statistical Office (1994) *Social Trends No. 24.* HMSO, London.

3 Gray-Donald KL, Payette H, Boutier V *et al.* (1994) Evaluation of the dietary intake of homebound elderly and the feasibility of dietary supplementation. *J American College of Nutrition* **13**:3:277–84.

4 Morgan DB, Newton HMV, Scharah CJ *et al.* (1986) Abnormal indices of nutrition in the elderly: a study of different clinical groups. *Age and Ageing* **15**:65–76.

5 Penfold P and Crowther S (1989) Causes and management of neglected diet in the elderly. *Care of the Elderly* **1**:20–2.

6 Granieri E (1990) Nutrition and the older adult. *Dysphagia* **4**:196–201.

7 Powers JS and Folk MC (1992) Nutritional concerns in the elderly. *Southern Medical Journal* **85**:**11**:1107–12.

8 Department of Health (1991) *Dietary Reference Values for Food, Energy and Nutrients for the United Kingdom. Report on Health and Social Subjects No. 41.* Report of the

Panel on Dietary Reference Values of the Committee on Medical Aspects of Food Policy. HMSO, London.

9 Department of Health (1970) *Interim Report on Vitamin D by the Panel on Child Nutrition – First Report by the Panel on Nutrition of the Elderly*. HMSO, London.

10 Ruberg RL (1984) Role of nutrition in wound healing. *Surgical Clinics of North America* **64**:**4**:705–13.

11 Cohen D (1994) Dementia, depression and nutritional status. *Primary Care* **21**:**1**: 107–19.

12 Abbasi AA and Rudman D (1994) Under-nutrition in the nursing home: prevalence, consequences, cause and prevention. *Nutrition Reviews* **52**:**4**:113–22.

13 Pronsky Z (1993) *Food Medication Interactions*. (8th edn). Food Medication Interactions Publishers, USA.

14 Morley JE and Miller DK (1992) Malnutrition in the elderly. *Hospital Practice* **27**:95–116.

15 Lavik MRH, Vandeberg H, Schrijver J *et al.* (1992) Marginal nutritional status among institutionalised elderly women as compared to those living more independently (Dutch Nutrition Surveillance System). *J American College of Nutrition* **11**:**6**:673–81.

16 Lavik MRHY, Schneider P, Hulshof K *et al.* (1992) Institutionalised elderly women have lower food intake than do those living more independently (Dutch Nutrition Surveillance System). *J American College of Nutrition* **11**:**4**:432–40.

17 Finn S (1992) Finn offers testimony on nutrition and the elderly. *J American Dietetic Association* **92**:**9**:1064–6.

18 Hene S (1993) Dietetic intervention in private residential care for the elderly. *Nutrition of Food Science* **6**:32–4.

19 Davies L and Knutson KC (1991) Warning signals for malnutrition in the elderly. *J American Dietetic Association* **91**:**11**: 1413–17.

20 Caroline Walker Trust (1995) *Eating well for older people. Report of an Expert Working Group*. Wordworks, London.

21 Mian LC, McDowell JA and Heaney LK (1994) Nutritional assessment in the elderly in the ambulatory care setting. *Nurse Practitioner Forum* **5**:**1**:46–51.

Further reading

Nutrition Advisory Group for Elderly People (NAGE) (1993) *Dietetic Standards of Care for the Older Adult in Hospital*. British Dietetic Association (BDA), Birmingham.

NAGE (1989) *Eating Through the 90s*. BDA, Birmingham.

NAGE (1993) *In the Minority Through the 90s*. BDA, Birmingham.

NAGE (1995) *Taking Steps to Tackle Eating Problems*. BDA, Birmingham.

Royal College of Nursing (1993) *Nutritional Standards and the Older Adult*. RCN, London.

CHAPTER 7

Anticipatory care of older people in the community

David Beales and Alistair Tulloch

The last 30 years have seen revolutionary changes in general practice, especially in such areas as preventive care of the newborn, hypertensive and diabetic patients. During this time anticipatory care of elderly people has, however, remained something of a backwater, despite mounting evidence of unrecognized health and socio-economic problems coupled with unmet patient needs.

What is wrong with conventional care of older people?

The inadequacies in this field are already well documented and can be summarized as follows:

- under-recognition of certain medical disorders, especially depression, dementia, urinary tract disorders, conditions of the feet, other disorders affecting mobility,[1] anaemia,[2] endocrine conditions,[2] physical abuse[3,4] and alcoholism[5]

- under-recognition of disability, especially due to sensory impairment[6]

- patients poorly informed about disability appliances, benefits, entitlements and other services leading to poor uptake of these resources[7,8]

- failure to recognize and manage the stress for carers, especially those managing highly dependent relatives or friends[9–11]

- poor health education of the elderly[12]

- poor standards of recording and information display in support of clinical care.[13]

In order to address these shortcomings a programme is needed that has clear objectives which seek to identify medical, social, functional and environmental problems much earlier and manage them (whenever possible) promptly.

In the light of these facts, in 1990 the Conservative government introduced a new general practice contract which, *inter alia*, required the primary care team to offer an annual check-up to patients aged 75 years or more.[14] This embraced a review of sensory functions, mobility, mental and physical status (including incontinence), social environment and use of medicine. Family doctors found that they were untrained in the organization of such a programme, and for some specific aspects of the work, such as the measurement of disability. Despite this they were offered no additional training and were given no guidelines on the organization of the programmes. Delegation of the work to other members of the primary care team was allowed freely, again without any requirements for training or supervision. The programme lacked flexibility and took little account of the diverse needs of people in old age. Worst of all, the system was introduced without any evaluation of its cost-effectiveness, or requirements for audit to be incorporated.

Family doctors, often unconvinced of the value of screening, viewed this poorly planned and ill-organized programme with scepticism as it merely served to confirm their prejudices.

It is however, essential especially in view of the sharply rising number of people aged over 75 years, that we devise a cost-effective system of care of older people which meets their needs earlier, keeps them active and independent for longer and enables them to live the best life possible. This chapter reviews the historical background, defines the objectives of care, analyses the controlled trials in this field and describes several ways of designing a programme to produce the optimum results. Such a programme will inevitably involve some form of screening which needs to be defined in this context. Screening has been described by the WHO as 'the search for unrecognised disease or defects',[15] whereas in this field the need to identify functional and socio-economic problems is equally important. For this, the term 'population scanning' would seem more appropriate to emphasize the broader canvas. However, we have continued to use the word screening since this is the term in current use.

Before reviewing the research work it is important to define the objectives of care among older people and these are summarized in Box 7.1.

Historical background

It was the pioneering Rutherglen Experiment in 1954[16] which first drew the attention of doctors to the fact that conventional community care was overlooking a variety of problems in the management of older people.

Despite this important finding, there was little evidence to suggest that general practitioners

Box 7.1: Objectives of care of older people

Interim goals

To control suffering

To prevent disease and its complications

To prevent or postpone crisis, hospital referrals, and institutional care

To maintain function and independence

To promote patient interest and socialization

To help maintain the person in the most acceptable and appropriate setting

To help old people face death and die with dignity

Ultimate aims

To enable old people to lead the best life open to them and to be able (whenever possible) to pursue their remaining aspirations

To prolong active life

To ensure that they have a 'good' death

(GPs) modified their methods of care subsequently to resolve this problem. Ten years later Williamson et al.,[17] in a survey of three practices in the Edinburgh area, reported that patients over the age of 65 years had an average of just over three disabling conditions, more than half of which were unknown to the family doctor, although many of these were treatable. This influential paper led many doctors to be more active in the care of older people. A number of these doctors published the results of their work usually based on various types of screening involving GPs, health visitors, nurses and volunteers.[18-21] The overwhelming majority of these studies reported unrecognized problems and unreported need. In a survey of 29 papers on screening by Alistair Tulloch, only three claimed to have found little or no health problems previously unknown.[22-24]

However, two important practical difficulties arise from this work – the burden generated for the primary care team, particularly at the outset, was considerable and the fact that no proper study of the benefits and cost-effectiveness of the programme has been completed to date. Blanket screening of all patients over the age of 65 years proved impractical – most practices of average size (roughly 2000 patients) have 300–350 people in this category, and the figure would be very much higher in retirement areas. Accordingly, patients surveyed tended to be over the age of 75 years but many people in this category were in good health, while the unrecognized need in those aged 65–70 years was scarcely negligible.

Barber and Wallis[25] estimated that thorough screening involved the primary care team in nine hours work per week for a practice of average size, while in the Bicester practice (Alistair Tulloch), the figure estimated was nearer eight hours at the onset and 6.5 hours in follow-up review; although this figure was slightly lowered, by a reduction in visiting, to just over six hours – still a significant increase in the workload of the primary care team.

The next change was to consider focusing on elderly people who were 'at risk' because they were more vulnerable than average to the effects of any of the following problems:

- progression, or complications of pre-existing chronic disease particularly causing mental impairment, behavioural problems, instability and immobility, a distinct increase in the risk of falls, incontinence, functional disability and social handicap

- inadequate financial resources

- loneliness, a state of mind not to be equated simply with lack of social contact

- inadequacy of support by relatives, neighbours and friends

- loss of domestic and social function, or reduced social contact and integration

- loss of independence, the ultimate fear for older people especially if it is likely to lead to institutional admission, due to any of the above problems.

However, identifying and managing 'at risk' patients is more complex in practice than it appears, although most care workers agree that those aged 85 years or more are in a high-risk group. However, while there is an elite cohort

Box 7.2: High-risk factors in the elderly

High risk

- advanced age

- recent discharge from hospital

- recent change of home, especially from another area

- divorce or separation

Medium risk

- recent bereavement

- living alone

- social class V

Relatively low risk

- lack of social contact

- childless

- never married

---

within this group of people who are remarkably fit, healthy and active for their age, there are at the same time some people aged 67–74 years who are significantly at risk. The study by Vetter et al.[26] has also confirmed that using an age for cut-off alone is inappropriate. Taylor et al.[27] having studied risk factors in old age, reported that high-risk factors can be classified as shown in Box 7.2.

It must be recognized that some older people have flexibility and adaptability which belies the effect of these conditions and merely to list such problems without taking account of this consideration can make such profiles actively misleading.

Barber and Wallis in Glasgow[28] developed a mini-item questionnaire to identify older people in need of care. The questions were as follows.

1 Do you live on your own?

2 Are you without a relative you could call on for help?

3 Do you depend on someone for regular help?

4 Are there days when you are unable to prepare a hot meal for yourself?

5 Are you confined to your home through ill-health?

6 Is there anything about your health causing you concern or difficulty?

7 Do you have difficulty with vision?

8 Do you have difficulty with hearing?

9 Have you been in hospital during the past year?

With a response rate of 81%, sensitivity of 0.95, specificity of 0.68 and a predictive value of 0.91 this proved to be an acceptable and effective sifting instrument. It was also estimated that it could reduce the workload of an assessment programme by one-fifth.

Thereafter, more comprehensive assessment questionnaires were used in some practices and examples of some of these are given in Appendix 1.

The next advance came from Freer[29] who recommended opportunistic screening when the patients came to consult their GP. He drew attention to the finding by Williams[30] that some 93% of people over the age of 75 years consult their doctors each year, while three studies[30–32] had shown that low-rate consulters were generally in good health. It is obviously wise to capitalize on a patient's attendance at surgery to collect relevant information on their health and functional status, and many family doctors find this a useful approach. However, since a thorough socio-medical assessment rarely takes less than 75 minutes of the time of the primary care team it is hard to see how this socio-medical assessment can be fitted into a busy surgery in its entirety. We therefore believe that the information collected opportunistically needs to be supplemented by assessment in an *ad hoc* clinic at the surgery, or by assessment in the home environment.

Tulloch[33] and Beales et al.[34] on the other hand have developed programmes for screening of all patients over the age of 75 years using volunteers to reduce the burden on the primary care team. Tulloch estimates that the volunteers spent about 4–5 hours per week on the work reduced to about three hours on follow-up, while he and the nurse or health visitor needed an additional 3–4 hours initially, reduced on the follow-up to three hours. The reduction in home visiting which resulted made the programme practical, and there was no evidence of an increase in the rate of consulting by older people as a result of the programme being established. McIntosh[35] has described a similar programme of which details are given in Chapter 8. The system is used in a number of practices in Scotland.

This covers the historical background to the introduction of the New Contract in 1990 which requires annual social and medical assessment of people aged 75 years or more.

Review of the evaluation studies of screening

As already stated there has been a variety of screening studies since 1954, the overwhelming majority of them showing unrecognized socio-medical problems. However, for an objective view of the value of screening we propose to rely on the main results of the randomized controlled trials done in this field (see Tables 7.1 and 7.2).

The first study by Tulloch and Moore[2] in patients aged over 70 years kept under screening and surveillance for two years, showed no effect on health or disability, but there was a rise in the number of institutional referrals and admissions. The most important finding however was that the duration of institutional bed days was reduced and the reduction was statistically significant. Then Row et al.[36] reported on patients aged 80 years or more who were screened and kept under review for 18 months. They found, in screened patients, a reduction of disability and in the number of institutional bed days. Neither finding was held to be statistically significant. Next Hendriksen et al.[37] reviewed patients aged 75 years or more over a period of three years. They found that in screened patients, contact with the primary care team, institutional admissions and use of social services were raised. However, the results found to be statistically significant were the reduction in emergency calls, duration of institutional care and mortality plus an increase in the use of home helps. Vetter et al.,[38] in a study of patients aged 70 years or more also found in screened patients a significant increase in institutional admissions and use of community services. In addition, one of the two practices involved reported a significant increase in the use of nursing, chiropody and home-help services. Finally, the death rate was reduced significantly in screened patients. Carpenter and Demopoulos[39]

Table 7.1: Results of randomized controlled trials reporting on the effectiveness of screening

	1979[2]	1983[36]	1984[37]	1984[38]	1990[39]	1990[40]	1992[41]	1993[42]
				Number of old people in the study				
	295	912	572	554	539	296	725	580
				Age range/duration of study				
	70+/2y	80+/18m	75+/3y	70+/24m	75+/3y	75+/20m	65+/3y	75–84/3y
Unrecognized disease								
System:								
1 CVS	+	+	–	–	–	–	–	–
2 MSS	+	+	–	–	–	–	–	–
3 CNS (& Sense Organs)	+	+	–	–	–	–	–	–
Effect on:								
1 health	0	–	–	–	–	–	–	0
2 disability	0	↓	–	0	0	–	–	–
3 quality of life	↑	–	–	↑	+	–	–	–
4 physical problems	–	–	–	–	–	0	–	–
5 anxiety	–	–	–	0	–	–	–	–
6 depression	–	–	–	0	–	–	–	–
7 ADL	–	–	–	–	0	–	–	0
Mortality	–	–	↓↓	↓↓⊗	0	0	↓↓	0
Patient:								
1 more health conscious	–	–	–	–	+	0	–	–
2 morale improved	×	–	–	–	–	↑↑	–	–
3 self-esteem increased	×	–	+	–	–	–	–	–
4 felt benefit of programme	×	–	+	–	–	–	–	–
5 kept independent for longer	×	–	–	–	–	–	–	–
6 well adapted to programme	+	–	–	–	–	+	–	–
7 falls reduced	–	–	–	–	++	–	–	0
8 change in subjective view of life	–	–	–	+	–	–	↑	0
9 favourably disposed to screening	+	+	+	–	+	–	–	–
10 did not find screening intrusive	×	–	+	–	–	–	–	–
11 co-operative	+	–	+	–	–	–	–	–
12 loneliness	–	–	–	–	–	++	–	–
13 emotion reaction	–	–	–	–	–	++	–	–
14 isolation	–	–	–	–	–	++	–	–
15 patient's overall rating of health employment	–	–	–	–	–	–	++	–

× impression positive change
↑ moderate, but not significant increase
↑↑ significant increase
↓ moderate, but not significant decrease
↓↓ significant decrease
+ positive, but not significant finding, or effect
++ significant positive finding, or effect
↓↓⊗ significant negative finding, or effect in one of two groups
0 no effect, or change
– not reviewed

Table 7.2: Results of randomized controlled trials reporting on the effectiveness of screening

	1979[2]	1983[36]	1984[37]	1984[38]	1990[39]	1990[40]	1992[41]	1993[42]
				Number of old people in the study				
	295	912	572	554	539	296	725	580
				Age range/duration of study				
	70+/2y	80+/18m	75+/3y	70+/24m	75+/3y	75+/20m	65+/3y	75–84/3y
Institutional referrals	↑	–	–	–	–	–	–	–
Institutional admissions	↑	–	↑	↑↑	–	0	↑	
Bed days institution care	↓↓	↓	↓↓	–	↓↓	–	↓↓	↓
Referral geriatric day hospital	–	–	–	–	↑↑	–	–	–
Attendance at day hospital	–	–	–	–	–	–	↓↓	–
Change of:								
1 contact with GPs	–	–	0	0	0	–	0⁺	–
2 contact with primary care team	–	–	↑	–	0	–	–	–
3 emergency calls	–	–	↓↓	–	–	–	–	–
4 domiciliary consultation with specialist	–	–	–	–	0	–	0	–
Use of community social services:								
1 raised	↑↑	–	↑	↑↑	↑	–	–	–
2 improved	×	–	–	↑	↑	–	–	–
Use of:								
1 physiotherapist	↑↑	–	–	↑↑	–	–	–	–
2 nursing	↑↑	–	–	↑↑⊗	0	–	–	–
3 chiropody	↑↑	–	–	↑↑⊗	–	–	–	–
4 meals-on-wheels	–	–	–	0	↑	–	–	–
5 home-helps	–	–	↑↑	↑↑⊗	↑	–	–	–
Volunteer screening effective	+	–	–	–	+	–	–	–
Important one person coordinates	–	–	+	–	+	–	–	–
Minor changes decisive	–	–	+	–	+	–	–	–
Programme cost-effective	–	*	**	–	*	–	–	□

× impression positive change
↑ moderate, but not significant increase
↑↑ significant increase
↑↑⊗ significant increase in one of two groups
↓ moderate, but not significant decrease
↓↓ significant decrease
+ positive, but not significant finding, or effect
0 no effect, or change
– not reviewed
* cost-effective
** highly cost-effective
□ not thought to be cost-effective
0⁺ GPs' hours, more consultations but fewer visits to surgery and significantly fewer home visits, thought to have produced a net reduction

in a study of patients aged 75 years or more over three years showed, in screened patients, no effect on disability or mortality but a significant reduction in duration of institutional care and an increase in the referral rate for day care. McEwan et al.[40] in a study of those aged 75 years or more over 20 months showed no effect on physical problems or mortality but found morale significantly improved, while loneliness and isolation were significantly reduced. The rate of institutional admissions was unchanged. Pathy et al.[41] reviewed patients aged 65 years or more over three years and in screened patients found a significant reduction in bed days of institutional care, attendance at day hospital and improvement in the patients' overall rating of their health. Finally van Rossum et al.[42] found, in screened patients only, a reduction in the duration of institutional care which was not statistically significant. However the difference was found to be statistically significant in a sub-group with perceived ill-health.

Discussion of results

The above results show that there is no consistent pattern in the findings of the controlled trials of screening reviewed. However this is scarcely surprising given the heterogeneous nature of elderly people in physical state, health, function, social and economic status. Also the studies themselves vary in their design, size, duration and indicators of outcome, while some deal with small numbers making it hard to draw firm inferences from the results.

The most promising finding however was the relative consistency of the reduction in duration of institutional care among screened patients. It was found in all of the six studies in which this indicator was used, although the difference was only statistically significant in four of them. If this finding were confirmed by a more powerful study it alone would make the exercise worthwhile. Very few patients want to end their days in a hospital or nursing home and such care is among the most expensive services in the National Health Service. Other findings made in the controlled trials suggest that there was still a fair amount of undiagnosed health problems and need especially in the cardiovascular, musculoskeletal

and nervous systems (including sense organs).[2,36] Screening does not appear to improve health significantly and the effect on disability and the death rate is uncertain over periods of up to three years. It does seem that rates of referral to day hospitals and institutional admissions are increased.

Other significant findings made in selected reports were that morale was improved[2,40] and patients felt less lonely, emotional and isolated.[40]

There was however no evidence to support the case raised by opponents of screening. Indeed emergency calls were reduced in one paper.[38] The rate of general practice consulting was not increased in four reports.[37–39,41] Patients did not find the screening intrusive[2,39] and only a tiny minority rejected this approach. The increased workload which was the primary concern among family doctors can be kept to manageable proportions by the use of volunteers.[2,34,39] It seems likely that screening will lead to an increase in the use of social services and one paper draws attention to the importance of one person coordinating the programme[37] while others emphasized that minor changes in health and function could be decisive in old age.[37,39]

With regard to cost-effectiveness, which was reviewed in four papers, the authors were convinced of its value in three cases[36,37,39] but the methods of measurement in all four studies were rather crude.

It is as yet uncertain as to how much can be achieved by screening and surveillance of the elderly but a research study is currently being run by the Medical Research Council which should provide the answer to important questions in this field:[43]

- what is the extent of unmet need in the community?

- can these problems be recognized by a brief questionnaire, or is a detailed questionnaire necessary?

- how effective is it simply to send a brief questionnaire to the patient through the post?

- if the brief questionnaire is to be administered, should this be done by a lay person or does it require a nurse?

- if a detailed questionnaire is used should this only be done in those positive on the brief questionnaire, or in every case?

- is a thorough assessment carried out by the primary care or geriatric team needed, and which team should undertake this work?

- how cost-effective is screening?

References

1 Williamson J (1981) The preventative approach in *The Provision of Care for the Elderly* (eds Kinaird J, Brotherstone JHF, Williamson J), Churchill Livingstone, Edinburgh.

2 Tulloch AJ and Moore V (1979) A randomised controlled trial of geriatric screening and surveillance in general practice. *J Royal College General Practitioners* **29**:355–9.

3 Hocking ED (1988) Miscare – a form of abuse of the elderly. *Update* **36**:2411–19.

4 Tomlin S (1992) *Abuse of elderly people: an unnecessary and preventable problem.* A public information report from the British Geriatrics Society, London.

5 Reid ALA, Webb GR, Hennrikus D *et al.* (1986) Detection of patients with high alcohol intake by general practitioners. *BMJ* **293**:735–8.

6 Hart CR and Burke P (1992) *Screening and Surveillance in General Practice.* Churchill Livingstone, Edinburgh, p. 263.

7 George J, Binns VE, Clayden AD *et al.* (1988) Aids and adaptations for the elderly at home: underprovided. *BMJ* **296**:1365–6.

8 Salvage AV, Jones DA and Vetter NH (1988) Awareness of and satisfaction with community services in a random sample of over 70s. *Health Trends* **20**:88–92.

9 Hicks C (1988) *Who cares: looking after old people at home.* Virago Press Ltd, Reading.

10 Leven E, Sinclair I and Gorbach P (1989) *Families, Services and Confusion in Old Age.* Gower Publishing Co. Ltd, Aldershot.

11 Jones DA and Vetter NJ (1985) Formal and informal support received by carers of elderly dependants. *BMJ* **291**:643–5.

12 Lucas S (1978) *Health Education in General Practice: an analysis of information and advice given by doctors in consultations with elderly patients.* Institute for Social Studies in Medical Care. (Unpublished.)

13 Cartwright A and Smith C (1988) *Elderly people, their medicines and their doctors.* Routledge, London.

14 Department of Health and Welsh Office (1989) *General Practice in the National Health Service: A New Contract.* Department of Health and the Welsh Office, February.

15 Wilson JMG and Jungner G (1968) *Principles and practice of screening for disease.* World Health Organisation, Geneva.

16 Anderson WF and Cowan NR (1955) A consultative health centre for older people. *Lancet* **2**:239–40.

17 Williamson J, Stokoe IH, Gray S *et al.* (1964) Old people at home: their unreported needs. *Lancet* **1**:1117–20.

18 Fairley HF (1967) Unrecognised disease among the elderly in general practice. *Practitioner* **199**:215–17.

19 Burns C (1969) Geriatric care in general practice. A medico-social survey of 391 patients undertaken by health visitors. *J Royal College General Practitioners* **18**:287–96.

20 Williams EI, Bennet FM, Nixon JV *et al.* (1972) Socio-medical study of patients over 75 in general practice *BMJ* **2**:445–8.

21 Currie G, MacNeill RM, Walker JG *et al.* (1974) Medical and social screening of patients aged 70 to 72 by an urban general practice health team. *BMJ* **2**:108–11.

22 Evans SM, Wilkes E and Dalrymple-Smith D (1970) Growing old: a country practice survey. *J Royal College General Practitioners* **20**:278–84.

23 Irwin WG (1971) Geriatric practice in the health centre. *Modern Geriatrics* **1**:265–6.

24 Freedman GR, Charlewood JE and Dodds PA (1978) Screening the aged in general practice. *J Royal College General Practitioners* **28**:421–5.

25 Barber JH and Wallis JB (1982) The effects of a system of geriatric screening and assessment on general practice workload. *Health Bulletin* **40/3**:125–32.

26 Vetter NJ, Lewis PA and Llewellyn L (1993) Is there a right age for case-finding in elderly people? *Age and Ageing* **22**:121–4.

27 Taylor R, Ford G and Barber JH (1983) *Research perspectives on ageing: the elderly at risk.* Age Concern, London.

28 Barber JH and Wallis JB (1980) A postal screening questionnaire in preventive geriatric care. *J Royal College General Practitioners* **30**:49–51.

29 Freer CB (1987) Consultation-based screening of the elderly in general practice: a pilot

study. *J Royal College General Practitioners* **37**:455–6.

30 Williams EI (1984) Characteristics of patients over 75 not seen during one year in general practice. *BMJ* **288**:119–21.

31 Ebrahim S, Hedley R and Sheldon M (1984) Low levels of ill-health among elderly non-consulters in general practice. *BMJ* **289**: 1273–5.

32 Goldman L (1984) Characteristics of patients aged over 75 not seen for one year in general practice. *BMJ* **288**:645.

33 Tulloch AJ (1992) Screening elderly patients. *The Practitioner* **236**:1022–6.

34 Beales D and Hicks E (1988) Volunteers help to detect unreported medical problems in the elderly. *The Practitioner* **232**:478–82.

35 McIntosh IB (1989) Comprehensive screening of over 75 year olds. *Geriatric Medicine* **198**:18–24.

36 Row OC, Bieren K, Bjornsen LE *et al.* (1983) *Eldreomoskorgens nye giv-et. Eskperiment med styrket innstats I primaertjenesten I Oslo.* Rapport Nr. 6 Oslo Gruppe for Helsetjenesteforskning.

37 Hendriksen C, Lund E and Stromgard E (1979) Consequences of assessment and intervention among elderly people: a three year randomised controlled trial. *BMJ* **289**:1522–4.

38 Vetter NJ, Jones DE and Victor CR (1984) Effect of health visitors working with elderly patients in general practice: a randomised controlled trial. *BMJ* **288**:369–72.

39 Carpenter GI and Demopoulos GR (1990) Screening the elderly in the community: controlled trial of dependency surveillance using a questionnaire administered by volunteers. *BMJ* **300**:1253–6.

40 McEwan RJ, Davison N, Forster DP *et al.* (1990) Screening elderly people in primary care: a randomised controlled trial. *British J General Practice* **40**:94–7.

41 Pathy MSJ, Bayer A, Harding K *et al.* (1992) Randomised trial of case-finding and surveillance of elderly people at home. *Lancet* **340**:890–3.

42 van Rossum E, Fredriks CMA, Philipsen H *et al.* (1993) Effect of preventive home visits to the elderly. *BMJ* **307**:27–32.

43 Bulpitt CG, Fletcher AF, Jones DA *et al.* (in progress) *Trial of the assessment and management of elderly people within the community.* Medical Research Council, London.

Further reading

Kennie DC (1993) *Preventive Care for Elderly People.* Cambridge University Press, Cambridge.

CHAPTER 8

The practical organization of screening and socio-medical assessment in old age

Iain McIntosh

Screening programmes raise mixed feelings among care workers, especially doctors, some of whom are strongly opposed to this approach often without having experience of the subject to any great degree. The author is, by contrast, firmly convinced of their value in improving patient care in old age and so are the editors of this book.

Screening older people is designed to identify and focus care on those thought to be 'at risk'. Thus it is hoped to achieve the objectives defined in earlier chapters. A further aim is more appropriate and more cost-effective provision of health care in old age – whether the service is purchased by health commissions or fundholding general practitioners (GPs).

Requirements for organization

Careful preparation and planning are essential and should include:

- defining clear objectives
- careful specification of the work to be undertaken
- design of suitable documentation
- training for all those involved
- plans for audit.

Once up and running, the organization and management of the programme needs to consider the following:

- identifying patients in the appropriate age group and particularly those known to be 'at risk'

- coordinating screening and follow-up

- on-going training programme for all health workers involved

- regular audit of the programme.

Detailed organization

Introductory meeting

It is best to start with an introductory meeting of all the health care professionals involved in elderly care, where the scope for a more active, anticipatory and interventionist programme is reviewed. Many practices are instigating practice profiling which offers an opportunity for multi-disciplinary review of the services already being provided. A SWOT analysis (strengths, weaknesses, opportunities and threats) is one tool useful in such a process. The programme must be seen as a worthwhile team project in which each worker has a great deal to contribute. All the workers should be given an opportunity to express their opinions and reservations which should be clearly addressed as far as possible. Staff also need to recognize that any process of change brings some anxieties. Opportunities for regular review, especially in the early stages, may help to allay fears.

Once agreement is reached, the objectives of the programme need to be defined clearly. An attempt should be made to estimate the additional workload depending on the size of the list and the percentage of patients aged over 75 years. In a well organized programme, approximately 1.25–1.5 hours of primary care team time per patient will be needed initially. The role and responsibilities of each worker must be clearly defined and the importance of co-operation and coordination of activities cannot be too strongly emphasized. An essential role is that of the coordinator, who needs a clinical background as it is they who will review the initial screening phase and identify those patients to be seen in the second phase. It may be appropriate to consider the appointment of a specially trained nurse or health visitor to work on this programme. Another major question is whether to use lay workers as in the Bicester and Phoenix models (see Appendices 1 and 3). The resource issues associated with the programme will need to be discussed at partnership level.

Design of questionnaire

Next it is vital to undertake detailed design of the questionnaires and forms to be used unless the practice decides to apply or modify forms used elsewhere. Some models are shown in the appendices. The administrative details need to be clarified, including the identification of patients, the two-phase process of screening – screening questionnaire and socio-medical assessment – including where and how the screening is to be offered, and follow up. Most practices will now have an age/sex register from which a listing of patients over the age of 75 can be produced stratified into those aged over 85, and those aged 75–84. From within this list, known 'at risk' patients can then be identified and approached first. Until the programme is established it will be necessary to prioritize patients to be approached, probably on a monthly basis. Whatever system is used it should be flexible enough to take account of predictable pressure points such as holidays and the unexpected – staff illness, periods of work overload, etc.

Computerization

The computer offers a range of services in this field not open to those using only manual systems. It facilitates the generation and updating of records, as well as analysis, recall, generation of clinic appointments and visiting lists, etc. A nominated clerk should be responsible for updating the age/sex register, ensuring input of data to the computer, producing patient tests, arranging clinics and visits. It is vital to enter the data promptly and to update it regularly, which is why a nominated clerk must be responsible for the work with a deputy when he or she is absent. Ideally, the practice manager will supervise this work and cajole or pressurize dilatory doctors into meeting their review commitments.

Training programme

Thereafter, a training programme must be organized for all members of the primary care team, including the doctors. Account needs to be taken of previous experience and knowledge as well as identifying the key skills needed, especially on assessment of disability and handicap. Emphasis will also be on good communication and on the importance of one person coordinating the programme, especially in more complex cases. Whilst multi-disciplinary training has many advantages in helping team members be clear about roles and responsibilities, there may also be a place for more detailed work with members of the team. For example, consideration will already have been given to the appointment of lay workers who may need more training. The training programme can involve workers from other agencies – social services or local voluntary groups who may have contact with the scheme or receive referrals. Such involvement is a good opportunity to help appreciate the perspective of others, whose basic approach may be different from members of the primary care team, as well as to educate them about the programme.

The Community Care Act has given social services a very important role in care of the elderly and their incorporation in the team is vital. They open the door to home-care provision and respite care and now have their own contractual obligations to older people to offer a needs assessment. This service was extended to carers from April 1996. Health care and social workers must try to find common ground in assessing medical and social needs, even if their basic approach is different. Regular contact and formal sharing of information (with due regard for confidentiality) as well as flexibility on both sides is vital.

In the course of the training, all staff should be briefed on the problems and needs of patients most often overlooked by conventional care and of the significance – especially in the very old – of paramedical problems in determining the quality of a patient's life. They should also be made aware of the strong functional orientation of the programme and of its emphasis on keeping older people independent for as long as possible. It is, in addition, vitally important for staff to recognize that care needs to be tailored to individual patient need.

Finally, staff need to be briefed carefully about the weekly multi-disciplinary care conference at which this work is discussed and reviewed to maintain co-operation and integration of activities. Care must be taken at these conferences to ensure that patient confidentiality is respected at all times.

'Screening' and socio-medical assessment

The initial screening by questionnaire can then be started, by post or administered by lay worker or nurse. It can be done in part opportunistically where the patient attends surgery, in an *ad hoc* clinic, or in the patient's home if he or she is unfit to visit the surgery, or if the home environment needs careful review.

The initial screening will then be supervised by the programme coordinator. Those patients identified as having significant disability or handicap will have a thorough medico-social assessment, usually carried out jointly by a doctor and nurse in a clinic or at the patient's home. If appropriate, the opportunity will be taken to give the patient health education on exercise, diet, environmental requirements, etc. Finally, a careful review of drug status will be undertaken. A profile of the patient's problems can then be completed in order of their importance and – to ensure that it is representative – a measure of the patient's adaptation to them needs to be incorporated. Management can be agreed by the team to meet the patient's needs. Care must be planned and delegated to team members as appropriate, one of whom should take prime responsibility for coordinating care. Finally, plans for review should be formulated to ensure that once problems are identified the effectiveness of intervention is monitored regularly.

Audit

Audit of the programme as a whole has to be built in at the planning stage. Key data include outline biographical details, functional and other assessment scores and action. Careful use of the practice computer can pay dividends at this stage.

Potential problems

In a sophisticated programme like this problems are sure to arise and, sadly, the most damaging is a prejudiced, inflexible attitude on the part of care workers, especially doctors, towards this approach. There is already evidence that some doctors have preferred to deal only with uncovered physical illness.[1,2] However, attitudes seem to be changing and the increasingly multi-disciplinary nature of primary care is bringing other perspectives to bear, in particular the social and emotional issues that can be addressed as well as maintaining function.

When any radical change of approach is introduced workers may feel threatened, especially if the programme involves new staff who may appear to be eroding their role and field of work. They are likely to be particularly suspicious of lay workers, those with limited training and 'outsiders' thought not to be like-minded, e.g. social workers. Equally, social workers may not appreciate the value of thorough medical review and diagnosis with appropriate treatment and may only see the need for home-care provision.

Many practices are already carrying a heavy workload these days and, if it is to be increased, extra staff provision will be vital especially to cover spells of illness and holidays. Sometimes assessment procedures differ, e.g. as between medical staff and social workers. These different approaches need to be explored; there will be differing needs depending on the agency but there is also likely to be scope for some stand-ardization.

Information systems

Attention has been drawn earlier to the need for carefully designed questionnaires and forms to be used if the programme is to be properly organized. A well-designed information system of this type should meet the following requirements:

- provides comprehensive cover of relevant data

- reflects the patient's physical, psychological, functional and socio-economic status

- provides data on support networks, therapy and service requirements and provision

- records system designed to express its message clearly with important data easily accessible

- computer input, audit and recall facilitated

- can be administered by health visitor, nurse or trained link worker.

Programme organization

Using the computerized age/sex register of those aged 75 years in the practice, a clerk can first generate a list of those patients in birth-date order. Patients thought to be at special risk (as defined earlier) are given priority and within the group those first seen tend to be the very old and the most highly disabled. Small cohorts are then selected in rotation for review by the geriatric health visitor (GHV) in special groups, in most cases at the surgery. When patients are unfit to be brought to the surgery or when the home envir-onment needs assessment they should be seen at home. The visits or consultations should always be carefully arranged in advance so that the patients are absolutely clear about the nature of the assessment and are able, if they want, to refuse the service. Part of the assessment can be done opportunistically when the patient is already having a consultation at the surgery.

The assessment itself is designed to review physical, psychological, social, environmental and economic factors and is particularly orientated to review of health and functional status plus early identification of dependency. Prior to seeing the patient the GHV will review the patient's file to establish what is already known on the above topics together with the patient's current therapy. The GHV will take the patient through the check-list (Appendix 2), covering the current social and health service use and the additional input required. The GHV will then review the patient's home environment, personal hygiene and diet. Finally, the GHV will assess the patient's capacity in activities of daily living with particular em-phasis on mobility, visual and auditory function and emotional status.

Activities of daily living are reviewed partic-ularly carefully. All these factors are scored and the scores are aggregated to reflect a patient's vulnerability. High scores returned in emotional, sleep and bereavement categories should trigger the use of BASDEC self-assessment cards or the Geriatric Depression Rating Scale to help uncover previously unsuspected depression. The nurse then administers the abbreviated mental test (AMT) to review cognition. Fears that this might distress the patient have not materialized. A high AMT score may indicate dementia and to estab-lish whether this is the case the clock-face test should be used. The patient is asked to enter the hour figures on an empty clock-face and then to draw in the clock hands for a specific time. Failure to do this reasonably accurately may support a provisional diagnosis of early dementia. Particular attention is paid to memory ' loss, especially for recent events. Thereafter the nurse reviews the therapy and the patient's compliance with advice with the aid of information from the computerized prescription printout. Anomalies are recorded and reported to the doctor.

Then the nurse checks the patient's weight, blood pressure and urine as well as testing sight and hearing. Some time is then spent with the patient on health education, covering topics like diet, exercise, home safety, disability benefits, etc.

Thereafter the doctor, armed with the above records, conducts a clinical assessment. This does not always involve a complete physical assessment, especially if the patient has had a recent physical check-up.

The GP will do 3–4 such assessments per week and the increase in workload is offset by a reduction in out-of-hours calls.[1] It may also reduce visiting and crisis intervention. These findings are again scored and the final total gives the primary care team a useful measure of a patient's vulnerability. Problems identified on screening and clinical assessment requiring management are reported to the appropriate health or social worker.

The data are also entered into a computer which helps generate patient recall, and facilitates planning and organization of the programme.

The programme, which is very popular with patients, enables the primary care team to identify and manage problems earlier and we believe that it keeps older people active for longer. In addition, the computerized database provides a valuable reservoir for audit and research.

Conclusion

Conventional care of old people in the community prior to 1990 was largely demand-led and there is plenty of evidence that it caused doctors to overlook health and social problems as well as patient needs. It is sometimes suggested that much of the research work in this field is now out of date and that standards of general practice have risen so much that little is being missed by the primary care team. This is certainly not confirmed by more recent studies. In 1990 Brown et al.[2] reported in a study of 20 practices, involving 331 patients aged 75 years or more, that just over 40% of the 484 problems found were unrecognized prior to screening. Reporting in 1997[3] they found that in a study of the same age group in 40 practices nearly half the patients assessed were found to have problems for which some action was taken. Thus the changes introduced under the New Contract in 1990 appear not to have resolved the defects of mainly demand-led care defined in Chapter 7. This is not surprising as they were untested, poorly planned and badly organized as well as being poorly implemented in many practices.[4] As a result, these measures are most unlikely to be cost-effective.

It is therefore vital for doctors to address the problems arising in community care of the elderly and to design programmes which will resolve them. The requirements for such a programme are:

- a recognition of the need for a new approach

- an awareness of the diversity of needs of older people

- clear objectives in care of the elderly

- a well-designed programme of anticipatory and clinical care

- flexible staff clearly aware of their roles and those of other members

- good records and clear-cut communication

- built-in audit

- appropriate modification of the programme as problems arise

- the need for one person to coordinate the programme.

The value of screening is, as yet, not properly established and we are not even sure at present how it should be designed and implemented. However, research suggests a variety of potential benefits, the most important of which is likely to be that reduction in institutional care may result from careful screening. If confirmed, this alone would make the exercise worthwhile. There are also subtle, but important, benefits from a well-run programme. Care is systematized and recording systems improved so that better monitoring of the patient is facilitated. Health education is also facilitated and patients tend to feel that a special interest is being taken in their welfare, which strengthens the doctor–patient relationship. As a result, it is popular with patients and their morale and self-esteem seem to be raised. This has been the experience of the author, although the scientific evidence to support claims of these subtle changes is not well established. Those who do not share this view will no doubt wish to advance alternative programmes to meet the shortcomings of conventional care documented earlier in the chapter.

The author and the sampled patients are firmly convinced that screening programmes improve care in their practices and patients nearly always welcome the special interest being taken in their health and welfare; although a small minority prefer not to have physical check-ups.

References

1 McIntosh IB, Young M and Stewart T (1988) General practice surveillance and management using a 2 year trained nurse. *Scot Med J* **33**:332–3.

2 Brown K, Williams EI and Groom L (1992) Health checks on patients aged 75 years and over in Nottinghamshire after the new GP contract. *BMJ* **305**:619–21.

3 Brown K, Best D, Groom L *et al.* (1997) Problems found in the over-75s by the annual health check. *Br J Gen Pract* **47**:31–5.

4 Tremellen J (1992) Assessment of patients aged over 75 years in general practice. *BMJ* **305**:621–4.

Further reading

McIntosh IB (1988) A general practice geriatric surveillance project. *Scot Med J* **33**:330–3.

McIntosh IB, Power K and Reed J (1993) Elderly people's views of annual screening assessment. *J Roy Coll Gen Practit* **43**:189–93.

Wilkinson C, Campbell A, McWhirter M *et al.* (1996) Standardisation of health assessments for patients aged 75 years and over. *Br J Gen Pract* **46**:307–8.

Young M and Chamove A (1989) Screening evaluation of the elderly. *Scot Med J* **9**:10–11.

CHAPTER 9

Health promotion and keeping fit in old age

Marion McMurdo

The word health is derived from the same root as 'hale' or 'whole', indicating that the concept of health concerns the whole person and their wellbeing. The World Health Organisation uses the following definition of health:

Health is a state of complete physical, mental and social well-being, not merely the absence of disease or infirmity.

In the eyes of many old people, however, health often equates with independence. An elderly individual may suffer from multiple medical problems, but so long as he/she is able to do the housework, he/she claims to be healthy.

Illness has been likened to an overflowing bath, and recent moves in the direction of health promotion have suggested that health professionals might be better employed turning off the taps rather than mopping the floor. This section of the chapter considers the range of health promotion practices in old age, and also highlights potential obstacles and pitfalls.

The scope of health promotion in old age

Health promotion in the elderly is designed to help old people feel better as well as lowering the risk of disease. The main means doctors have

of preventing disease and promoting health is by offering or recommending services such as:

- counselling

- screening

- immunization.

In each of these, there is a need for partnership with the patient and clarification of goals in deciding on the best approach.

Health promotion also attempts to modify the environment in which old people live, for example, by providing information about available financial benefits. Social and environmental factors, such as poor housing and poverty, are major contributors to ill-health at all ages, although modification of these may be beyond the scope of the doctor.

Primary care is seen as a key setting for health promotion because four out of five people have annual contact with their general practitioners (GPs). Primary service health care workers also enjoy high status amongst the general public, and this credibility can be exploited to influence behaviour. Hospital doctors, however, for too long have been regarded as fulfilling only a specialist role in service and education, yet hospital doctors also have opportunities and responsibilities to educate the public. Hospital physicians have an important role in implementing the target set

Box 9.1: Health of the Nation targets for older people

- Coronary heart disease (CHD) and stroke:
  - to reduce the death rate for CHD in people aged 65–74 years by at least 40% by the year 2000
  - to reduce the death rate from stroke in people aged 65–74 years by at least 40% by the year 2000
- Cancer:
  - to reduce the death rate for lung cancer by at least 30% in men under 75 and 15% in women under 75 by 2010
- Mental illness:
  - to improve significantly the health and social functioning of mentally ill people
  - to reduce the overall suicide by 15% by the year 2000
- Accidents:
  - to reduce the death rate for accidents among people aged 65 and over by at least 33% by 2005

---

out in the Health of the Nation document (see Box 9.1).

Is it too late to promote health in old age?

Health promotion has been pursued with little enthusiasm in old age for a variety of reasons. Some health care workers believe that 'you can't teach an old dog new tricks' and that habits of a lifetime will already have wrought their irreversible havoc. This belief is wrong, certainly as far as cigarette smoking, exercise and treating high blood pressure are concerned. Another barrier is the belief of many older people themselves that a decline into old age is inevitable and that given their advanced years, the doctor might have more promising material on which to pursue his health promotion activities.

Autonomy refers to a person's capacity to choose freely for themselves and direct their own lives. Old people are particularly vulnerable to attacks on their autonomy, and in the recent past, many doctors were extremely paternalistic, especially towards the elderly. There is also a danger that relatives may take decisions on behalf of the old person, believing that 'they know best'. Respecting the wishes of the individual older person can be difficult for the more zealous health promoters. Persuasion should not be undue and the older individual's autonomy should be respected so that the final decision rests in their own hands. A good life necessitates risk-taking and in old age this is certainly the case.

Counselling

Many old people are socially isolated and have no living relatives. To help old people make decisions about lifestyle changes it is often useful for them to have a helper, adviser or carer with whom they can discuss the changes. A GP is particularly well placed to advise on lifestyle compared with other health professionals, because of the respect that the average person still has for their family doctor, but nurses and health visitors are sometimes equally well placed to provide this service.

Cigarette smoking

Many old people continue to smoke, and there is good evidence that the health risks associated with smoking continue into old age. The increased incidence of coronary thrombosis and lung cancer is well documented but additional smoking-related problems for elderly subjects are peripheral vascular disease, weight loss, functional decline and the increased fire risk that older people pose to themselves and others.

Even lifelong smokers who give up in old age should experience a reduction in mortality from coronary artery disease, lung cancer, pneumonia and influenza. Cigarette smoking is tackled less consistently in later life than in younger groups on the erroneous assumption that it will already have done its harm. Methods that have been shown to be effective in assisting people to give up tobacco use include simple physician counselling and the use of nicotine substitutes. Only one-third of smokers acknowledge having been advised by their doctors to stop smoking, but most claim they would make a serious attempt to do so if their doctor recommended it.

At the same time, it has to be recognized that there are patients, especially the very old, to whom smoking is one of the few pleasures left in life. It may be inappropriate in some cases to pressurize such patients too zealously to forsake smoking.

Alcohol

High or even moderate alcohol intake is associated with an increased risk of hip fracture, partly due to alcohol making a fall more likely. Between 2 and 10% of pensioners are problem drinkers, and characteristically present with gastrointestinal problems, trauma, neglect or confusional states. The CAGE questionnaire has been shown to discriminate successfully between older people with and without drink-related problems (see Box 9.2). Counselling should focus responsibility for the decision not to drink where it belongs: with the patient. Older people should be encouraged to replace drinking alone or in a public house with social activities, or the company of those who drink modestly or not at all. This may include self-help groups or voluntary community interests trying to persuade such people to change their lifestyles in this field.

Box 9.2: CAGE questionnaire

Have you ever felt you should **C**ut down on your drinking?

Have people **A**nnoyed you by criticizing your drinking?

Have you ever felt bad or **G**uilty about your drinking?

Have you ever had a drink first thing in the morning to steady your nerves or to get rid of a hangover (**E**ye-opener)?

Exercise

Participation in regular exercise declines with age for a variety of reasons which will be discussed in more detail below. The hazards associated with immobility in old age are legion and include muscle wasting and contraction, osteoporosis, pressure sores, deep venous thrombosis, heart disease, depression and bronchopneumonia. There is no doubt, however, that the health benefits of exercise outweigh the risks at all ages. Elderly people require the encouragement and support of their doctors to resume exercise after a prolonged period of inactivity. Rehabilitation after illness and injury is also particularly important in the elderly and should be actively pursued.

Screening

The objective of screening is the early diagnosis of presymptomatic, unrecognized or unreported disease. Screening differs from traditional medicine in that it attempts to detect disease *before* an individual seeks medical advice and often before symptoms are evident or their significance recognized by the patient. Therefore, screening carries a considerable ethical responsibility, as it is only justifiable when seeking disorders in which earlier intervention should improve outcome (see Box 9.3). Opinions on the value of screening remain mixed, particularly in general practice. Consumer-led enthusiasm for screening has brought about the introduction of a contractual obligation for GPs to assess people over 75 years of age annually, despite a lack of clear evidence that such practices are effective.

Sensory and functional impairments

Most GPs focus on assessing visual acuity, hearing ability, dental condition and locomotor activity. Poor vision and hearing are common in later life, and may contribute to social isolation and confusion. Corrections of such disabilities can make an important contribution to quality of life. Support should also be given to the family or carer to help them cope, to reduce stress and to recognize their particular needs.

Box 9.3: Principles of screening

For screening to be effective for the condition or disease:

- the condition should be an important health problem

- there should be an accepted treatment for those with the disease

- there should be a recognizable early, or presymptomatic phase

- treatment of the disease in the early stage should be of more benefit than in the later stage

- there should be a suitable test which is acceptable to the patient

- the chance of physical or psychological harm to those screened should be less than the chance of benefit

- the cost of the screening should be balanced in relation to the benefit it provides.

Source: Wilson JMG and Jungner G (1968) *Principles and practice of screening for disease.* World Health Organisation, Geneva.

Blood pressure measurement

After a period of uncertainty, it is now clear that treating high blood pressure in old age is worthwhile, as it is associated with a reduction in deaths from stroke and cardiovascular events. This applies to both diastolic and isolated systolic hypertension. The increased risk of side-effects from antihypertensive therapy in the elderly is well known, and should be borne in mind as they may affect quality of life.

Immunization

Tetanus toxoid

Even though tetanus is uncommon in developed countries, prevention can be justified in elderly people because 60% of reported cases occur in pensioners. There is also a low prevalence of protective levels of serum anti-toxin in the older community. The routine immunizing schedule for older people is three doses, and a booster dose every ten years.

Influenza vaccine

Although rates of influenza-like illness in the older community are low, the high associated rates of complication and death justify preventive vaccination in high-risk groups. Annual vaccination with the current vaccine is recommended for high-risk older people, particularly those with cardiac or respiratory disease. Vaccinations of residents in long-stay hospital wards, nursing and residential homes is also recommended, although questions remain about the efficacy and ethical wisdom of such a sweeping approach.

Keeping fit

Preventing disability and dependence is the goal of all professionals involved in the care of elderly people. In recent years it has become accepted that many age-related changes that were once assumed to be solely the result of the ageing process are partly the result of disuse. This important distinction has revolutionized attitudes towards ageing, and offers the attractive prospect of postponing the 'decline' into old age, which was once considered to be inevitable. This section highlights the importance of physical fitness in old age, and provides guidance on how to motivate old people to exercise regularly.

Physical fitness

The common attributes of physical fitness include strength, stamina and suppleness. The component that is regarded as the 'gold standard' for fitness is aerobic capacity, or as it is measured in the physiology laboratory: maximal oxygen uptake. In practical terms, the better the aerobic capacity, the fitter the person and the less is the displacement of pulse, respiratory rate and other relevant variables from their resting levels when he/she performs work. The fitter the person, the less the body is disturbed by work, and the more quickly it returns to the resting state when the work is finished.

For a young adult, a loss of fitness will reveal itself only if the person is required to undertake some strenuous activity, for example playing a game of squash. He or she will however, have ample reserve capacity to cope with daily activities without difficulty. A lack of fitness does not impinge on the ability to conduct daily life. In stark contrast, the old person lacks the reserve capacity of his young counterpart, and so is precariously close to a point where a minor additional decline in muscle strength may render everyday activities impossible, or at least requiring such near-maximal effort as to be unpleasant to perform. So loss of fitness in old age may tip the balance between dependence and independence.

Habitual activity patterns in old age

There is little doubt that most adults in developed countries are woefully inactive. One survey from the US showed that 30% of adults had undertaken no exercise in the four weeks preceding the interview. Self-reported physical activity declines with increasing age, although many older people regard involvement in gardening and walking as exercise. The vigour of these activities is likely to be variable, adding to the difficulty of gaining a true pattern of activity levels in old people. Nonetheless, despite increasing survival times in post-retirement, 53% of a random sample of pensioners in Nottinghamshire reported no leisure physical activity of any sort.

Barriers to exercise

The barriers reflect the culture of old age in our society today, with its misconceptions about ageing, not least among the elderly themselves.

Expectation of society

Many people regard old age as a period of decline in which activity should be gradually reduced. Thus pensioners are advised to 'slow down', and 'put their feet up' as a reward for their years of toil. It is common practice for those approaching retirement to be moved to less physically demanding jobs. This is compounded by some well-intentioned relatives who assume cleaning and shopping chores, and actually hasten the onset of dependency. Undoubtedly some inappropriate social care encourages dependency and promotes helplessness.

Effects of disease

Diseases of the central nervous system, such as Parkinson's disease and stroke, are common in old age, and together with osteoarthritis often interfere with activity levels and mobility.

Ageing process

There is an age-related decline in skeletal muscle strength from around the fifth decade, although the rate varies from person to person. Low muscle mass means that each unit of muscle tissue is responsible for the support and movement of a greater proportion of the total mass. Thus muscles must exert a greater force, working closer to their maximum capacity and the onset of fatigue is hastened.

Lack of information

Many old people are unaware that exercise is a healthy and appropriate activity throughout life. Some who do wish to resume exercise need guidance on what constitutes healthy activity and how to get started. A lack of local facilities, transport problems and concerns about pre-existing medical conditions can all be obstacles.

Access and availability of facilities

A lack of transport, or poor timing of sessions for people who want exercise by swimming can all play a part in discouraging the elderly from taking exercise.

Box 9.4: Benefits of exercise in old age

- **Cardiovascular**
  - low blood pressure
  - improves lipid profile
  - reduces heart attack risk

- **Musculoskeletal**
  - improves joint flexibility
  - strengthens muscles
  - improves endurance
  - slows bone loss in osteoporosis
  - may improve balance

- **Psychological**
  - improves the quality of sleep
  - improves mood
  - lessens anxiety
  - makes participant 'feel good'

- **Functional activity**
  - improves functional status
  - may postpone the onset of dependence
  - makes day-to-day tasks easier

How much exercise is needed?

The benefits of exercise in old age are well established (see Box 9.4), so it is important to know how much exercise is required for health. The formal approach advocated by exercise scientists in recent decades has recommended specified intensities, durations and frequencies of exercise. This was driven by the notion that a minimum exercise intensity was required to achieve physical fitness. Such methods have led to the mistaken belief that unless a specified and substantial dose of exercise is achieved, there are no benefits or health gains. Evidence is now accumulating, however, that total energy expenditure rather than exercise intensity is the key factor. This supports a more linear dose-response relationship between exercise and health and functional benefits. This dose-response relationship is good news for the sedentary and the elderly. The public health message should be 'Doing a little exercise is better than doing none, and, to a degree, more is better than less'.

Continuous exercise is not necessary to achieve a training effect, as three 10-minute walks during the day have the same impact on physical fitness as one 30-minute walk. This type of approach is less intimidating and easier to follow than prescription of a continuous session. Indeed, if sedentary people accumulated 30 minutes of walking per day, they would attain clinically significant health benefits. Another important point is that it does not matter what type of exercise is performed: sports, exercise classes, golf, swimming, gardening and walking the dog are all beneficial. If additional energy expenditure consistently occurs, then improvements in health and fitness will ensue.

Safety during exercise

Safety is a key consideration when advocating exercise for older people. As old people tend to be less ambitious exercisers, both traumatic and over-use injuries occur less frequently than in younger counterparts. Means of avoiding musculoskeletal injury are given in Box 9.5. Warning symptoms during exercise include undue breathlessness, chest pain or dizziness. If, however, an activity is not provoking symptoms, it is very unlikely to be doing harm. Probably the most damaging phrase that has come to be associated with exercise in recent years is 'no pain, no gain'. This dangerous philosophy exhorts a mindless, competitive edge and is the cause of innumerable sporting injuries to people of all ages. It has no place in a strategy of pleasurable, lifelong physical activity.

One of the most remarkable aspects of research on exercise in the elderly has been the

Box 9.5: Factors contributing to musculoskeletal injury

Failure to warm-up adequately

Violent exercising, especially twisting

Over-doing it, i.e. exercising beyond the point of pleasant fatigue

Exercising on a hard, or uneven, surface

Wearing shoes with inadequate heels and poor ankle support

Source: Shephard RJ (1987) *Physical Activity and Ageing.* Croom Helm, London.

---

virtual absence of reports of serious complications. Cardiac rehabilitation programmes which enrol many patients over 65 years of age with known coronary artery disease, also report few major complications. In their concern for safety, it is easy for the health professional to lose sight of the fact that exercise is a normal, reasonable, health-enhancing behaviour. Thus exercise should be viewed as safe for most older adults.

Motivation

Sadly it is too often the case that the health professions are more conservative than the older person when it comes to providing exercise advice. To their shame, doctors have devoted too much of their energies to identifying reasons why old people should not exercise, and too little to why they should. Undue insistence on preliminary screening implies danger and can extinguish motivation. Advice should be simple and positive (see Box 9.6).

Conclusion

Throughout life, the health benefits of regular exercise far outweigh the hazards. Exercise confers social and psychological as well as physical benefits, and may help to counteract the isolation that can accompany later life. The most compelling argument for older people to keep fit is that doing so is a means of postponing physical dependency and prolonging active life

Box 9.6: Advice to older people on exercise

* Find an activity you enjoy
* Start slowly
* Gradually build up the amount you do
* Even small amounts of exercise can be good for you
* Exercising with a friend or in a group is more fun than on your own
* Walking is ideal exercise
* Try to build exercise into your daily routine, then it is less easily forgotten
* Exercise should leave you feeling slightly exhilarated, but not exhausted, so always exercise within your own level of comfort

expectancy. Old people should be informed that exercise is good for you regardless of age, and that they have the most to gain from exercise and the most to lose from inactivity.

Further reading

Kennie DC (1993) *Preventive Care For Elderly People*. Cambridge University Press, Cambridge.
Muir Gray JA (1985) *Prevention of Disease in the Elderly*. Churchill Livingstone, Edinburgh.

CHAPTER 10

Community nursing and primary care

Kate Saffin

This chapter reviews the contribution that community nursing can make to the care of elderly people in general practice, discusses their role within and associated with the primary care team and describes in more detail some of the specialist work each group undertakes. It also addresses some of the conflicts faced in teamwork, both within the primary health care team (PHCT), and more widely.

The PHCT has been a central plank of government health policy for more than a decade despite a lack of objective evidence for the clinical effectiveness of teamwork. Broadly speaking, while there is widespread support for the notion of primary care teams there are also concerns. Friction can be caused by poor communication, concern with status and poor or unclear role definition, especially as teams get larger.

However, few elderly patients have health needs so straightforward that only one service or health professional is needed to address them so collaborative working is essential. Good teamwork can offer a breadth of skills and knowledge, delegation to the most appropriate person and better care. However, teams do not simply happen, they need to be developed and supported. The challenge for PHCTs is to create structures that support joint working, avoid duplication and promote good care for patients.

Community nursing

Castledine (1996) describes the community as having eight areas of nursing specialism:[1]

1 general practice nursing

2 community mental health nursing

3 community mental handicap/learning disabilities nursing

4 community children's nursing

5 public health nursing – health visiting

6 occupational health nursing

7 community nursing in the home

8 school nursing.

There are also an increasing number of specialist nurses who may be based in the community or within the acute service, such as continence advisers, stoma care nurses and palliative care nurses.

It is a range that has grown up in an *ad hoc* way over the last hundred years. This growth has not always been straightforward. Twinn describes the internal and unhelpful conflicts in nursing as well as the policy framework that has resulted in fragmented nursing services in the community.[2] She discusses the development of the main specialisms in community nursing. From this one can identify three separate strands, each with a different philosophical base to their development and practice:

1 health visitors and district nurses with their origins in the nineteenth century public health movement

2 psychiatric and mental handicap nurses whose service grew out from hospitals

3 practice nurses, whose growth has been a direct response to government policy on primary care over the last ten years.

She argues that further inconsistencies occur in the preparation of practitioners for the community where health visitors require a statutory registrable qualification and other disciplines do not, leading to an implicit hierarchy. There are now attempts to deal with these historical divisions by joint training at foundation level.

All community nursing disciplines share certain underlying principles:

• supporting patients or clients in their own community

• encouraging independence

• acting as resource for the patient and their carers

• preserving confidentiality

• liaising with other professionals working with the same client or patient

• assessment and provision of care within their field

• health promotion; planned and/or opportunistic.

The skills that all the above disciplines share in common are those of assessment, planning and delivery of nursing care in settings including the patient's own home, residential homes, health centres, surgeries and community hospitals.

All will be registered nurses, many with additional qualifications for working in the community. Those without such specialist preparation are likely to be working at staff nurse grades as part of a team, supervised and supported by a senior nurse.

Nursing in the PHCT

Overview

Reid and David (1994) describe four different organizational models, each working well within its own setting, concluding that there is no ideal or model PHCT.[3] Common to all models is that the health workers involved will be providing services to a population defined by the practice list.

The core team will vary from practice to practice but most would accept that general practitioners (GPs), nurses (district nurses, health visitors, practice nurses) and midwives are included. Secretaries and receptionists also have an important part to play. In large group practices other health care professionals such as specialist nurses, dietitians, chiropodists, physiotherapists and occupational therapists may be included. In other, often inner-city areas, GPs remain isolated from colleagues and the PHCT may exist in name only.

In addition there are the nurses (and others) who work with a wider population than one practice list and who form an 'extended' team. These include community psychiatric nurses, school nurses and the professions allied to medicine. Recent additions to some teams have been services such as counselling and physiotherapy purchased by fundholders and the introduction of practice based, but independent, complementary therapies.[4]

Practice nursing

There were nurses working in general practice as early as 1910 but practice nursing as a distinct discipline was established following the General Practitioners Charter in 1966. Growth was slow over the next ten years but has been rapid since 1984, especially since the 1990 GP contract.

As a discipline, practice nursing has grown haphazardly, responding to the changing needs of general practice, with nurses extending their role to include monitoring care for elderly people with chronic conditions, such as diabetes or hypertension. Many practices managed the contractual obligation to offer an over 75-year-old health check by using the practice nurse, making her the central health professional in anticipatory care. This extended role could lead to much more joint co-operation with community nurses including home visiting and the implementation and monitoring of care plans for those with severe disability. Jones (1996) reports that in 1992 'half of older people had consulted a practice nurse in a 12 month period'.[5]

Unlike their colleagues in district nursing and health visiting, practice nurses are employed by the practice rather than an NHS trust. Many value the independence of working for GPs, although there are concerns about adequate time for training and professional support. Most health authorities (now merged with the former Family Health Services Authorities (FHSAs)) now employ practice nurse advisors to oversee education and professional development.

District nursing

District nurses provide nursing care at home. Whilst they are available to the whole practice population, the majority of their work is with elderly people. The emphasis of their work is in physical health problems, whether acute or chronic.

A report in 1991 reviewed the workload of nurses in three areas, and concluded that much could be delegated to less highly qualified nurses.[6] The majority of district nurses now work in teams comprising qualified district nurses (G grade), staff nurses (RN without post-registration training – usually D or E grade) and nursing assistants.

The Community Care Act has also had a fundamental impact on district nursing. The Act has shifted responsibility for much of the personal care traditionally provided by district nurses to care assistants. The line between nursing and social care now falls between the often nebulous concepts of 'social' personal care and 'nursing' personal care which can necessitate much time-consuming negotiation as to who does what.

Overall this has resulted in a fundamental change in the work of the district nurse who is now carrying out less personal hygiene care, and more assessment and complex care. While many have concerns about the changes, especially the quality of home care available to the elderly (now purchased by social services, either in-house or from private agencies), many find great satisfaction in being able to support more people with complex or palliative care needs at home.

Health visiting

The origins of health visiting lie in maternal and child welfare. However, many are now expanding their role, or specializing, to work with older people, usually in anticipatory care, such as screening and health education. The principles of health visiting, namely: the search for health needs, the stimulation of an awareness of health needs, the influence on policies affecting health and the facilitation of health enhancing activities, are as applicable to older people as they are to young families. Their work with older people on a day-to-day basis may include individual and group work through home visiting, working with groups and liaison with other agencies.

Nursing in community teams

Community psychiatric nursing (CPN)

The community psychiatric nurse will be a registered mental nurse; most will also have undertaken a further nine-month post-registration training in community psychiatric nursing, although this additional training is not mandatory.

The organization of the CPN service varies from area to area. In most districts, services for elderly people are provided by CPN nurses working solely with this age group. The developing model is for CPN nurses to work in multi-disciplinary teams, including geriatricians, occupational therapists and others. Such teams may be hospital or community based.

Like all community nurses, the CPN nurse initially assesses the patient and their situation. From there the care plan may include interventions such as psychological therapies, case management (coordinating and monitoring a care package) or monitoring psychotropic medication.

Community psychiatric nursing services specifically for elderly people developed against a background of increasing emphasis on community care and a policy to run down long-stay psychiatric hospitals. Their work increasingly supports people with dementia – and their carers – in the community. Depression too is a common psychiatric disorder among older people and may be under-detected and under-treated. The CPN nurse has much to offer in psychological therapies to this group.

The main concern of CPN nurses in relation to the PHCT is maintaining contact. A CPN nurse may be community or hospital based, but either way he or she may cover a large geographical area and need to liaise with several PHCTs. Fundholding has brought further uncertainties, as different practices purchase different levels of service.

Professions allied to medicine

Although the focus of this chapter is community nursing, there are a significant number of others contributing to the health care for elderly people. These include physio- and occupational therapists, podiatrists, dietitians and speech therapists. Podiatry is the service most commonly used by older people (apart from the GP) with 8% seeing one within any month (but 22% consulting within a three-month period) whereas only 4% have seen a district nurse and less than 1% a health visitor.[5] Occupational therapists are an unusual group in that most working in the community will be employed by the local authority with a particular responsibility for equipment and adaptations to the home. Those employed by the health service are likely to be found in day hospitals providing rehabilitation services.

Developing teamwork

There are tensions between professional autonomy and team working. Whilst the concept of team care is generally accepted, the guarding of professional boundaries and an increasing trend towards specialization may make it unworkable. However, at the same time there are innovative practices developing integrated nursing teams where there is a blurring of professional boundaries and a greater flexibility in working practices. Social-work links with practice teams add to integrated team working. However, there can be conflicts of loyalty for the primary care team members employed by a trust for whom the GP is a 'customer'. This can lead to a sense of being pulled in several directions at once and needs careful management if it is not to become destructive.

Communication is recognized to be the key to making teamwork effective. Establishing and maintaining links within and without a team is a time-consuming business and there are no short cuts. It helps if the members of the PHCT are based in the same building, and can meet face-to-face frequently – formally and informally. For those working in the wider community team, there needs to be arrangements by which they are able to meet regularly with the PHCTs in their area plus mechanisms to enable speedy contact when necessary.

Waine (1992) claims that 'confidentiality is often the altar on which effective communication is sacrificed'.[7] He criticizes the current practice of separate record keeping and suggests that a shared system must be 'seriously considered'. He does not, however, go as far as suggesting that this should be a patient-held record – the obvious place for the record to be if it is to be available to all who work with the patient. Communication can also be improved by greater understanding of roles. Some aspects of medical and nursing education are amenable to sharing, at both pre- and post-registration levels. Within the PHCT, a shared approach to service planning and needs assessment has proved to be a practical way to explore common goals and understanding.

The patient as co-worker

Most older people are fit and well with only a quarter (28%) assisted by one or more services each month;[5] although the introduction of the over-75 years health surveillance means that, in theory at least, all older people have contact with the PHCT every year.

Historically there has been a power imbalance between professional and patient. Latterly there is a greater emphasis on the needs and wishes of relatives and carers and the phrase 'working in partnership' is often heard. However it is a complex and difficult concept, not an easy solution. It requires not only changes in professional practice but also in public expectation.

The changes in provision following the Community Care Act have been felt by elderly people in terms of provision, cost and who arrives on their doorstep. They are no longer likely to receive any service if their only need is household help or assistance with bathing. If the personal care they need is deemed to be 'nursing' it will be free; if 'social' there will be a charge (which may be a fixed charge or means tested). The carer may be an employee of the NHS trust, social services or a private agency.

The Carers (Recognition & Services) Act 1995 specifies carers' entitlement to assessment. One hopes it will raise awareness and improve services, although carers' groups are concerned that without adequate resources little will change.

Most district nurses now keep their nursing records in the home, and carers are encouraged to read them, however there is little evidence that they write in them or use them when going to hospital or the GP. This is an area ripe for development which could provide a valuable tool in coordinating care.

For the patient, the role of the GP following discharge has been described akin to that of a border guard:[8]

> ... passing them back, in a familiar language, to a world, which while familiar, they had nevertheless partially forgotten and to which they had to adjust. Moreover the doctor as border guard could introduce them to the benefits of being home, and the resources available in the community.

It could be argued that there are others – nurses, social workers and volunteers who could 'introduce them to the benefits of being home, and the resources available in the community'. However, the patients in the study were emphatic about the importance of seeing the doctor (which few had). This result was replicated by Beales in a descriptive study of patient's experience after a hip fracture.[9] Only 19% of patients had received a planned visit from the GP at 28 days post-discharge, with a further 19% having a visit on request.

'Knowledge is power' is an oft repeated maxim. Parker and Beales found patients were often unaware of services available to them.[10] They conclude that general practice could be an ideal base for a helpline. There are now many alternatives to the traditional leaflet, such as videos, audio cassettes and computer-based interactive systems.

Case history

Mrs Clark is 84 and lives alone. She has been fit and active until a fall in which she fractured her hip.

Discharge planning begins in hospital with an assessment by the social worker and her named nurse on the ward. They conclude that she is likely to need ongoing support and so arrange a case conference to ensure that the care package is as comprehensive as possible. It is attended by the ward staff, the geriatrician, the physio- and occupational therapists and the district nurse who has discussed her medical history with the GP and with the practice nurse (who saw her recently for her annual over-75 check). The planning for her discharge includes a home visit accompanied by the occupational therapist who assesses her ability to cope at home and arranges for a stair rail to be fitted, blocks to raise her usual chair to a suitable height and a raised toilet seat. Ongoing rehabilitation is arranged via the local day hospital.

Following her discharge the district nurse visits and having assessed her feels the wound is not healing as well as it might. She arranges for the staff nurse to visit and redress the wound every two days and reviews regularly until it heals.

The hospital social worker has arranged a package of care that includes a care assistant visiting each morning to help Mrs Clark with personal care and dressing. Mrs Clark had assured her carers that a neighbour would do her shopping. Some weeks later the care assistant becomes concerned that there is very little food in the house and discusses the situation with the social worker. He visits to reassess and feels Mrs Clark may be depressed. He decides to increase the home-care on a temporary basis to support Mrs Clark while he contacts the PHCT to discuss the problem.

He meets with the district nurse and GP during his regular weekly visit to the practice. After some discussion about possible approaches the GP offers to visit as she feels a medical review may be necessary. She too finds Mrs Clark to be depressed but suggests referral to the CPN nurse rather than medication at this stage.

Over the next few months the CPN nurse works with Mrs Clark as well as liaising with the PHCT and social services. This results in a package of care that includes regular review of her needs with an appropriate mix of help and encouragement to regain her independence.

Conclusion

The story of Mrs Clark is a somewhat idealized picture of how services can work. It also illustrates the variety of nurses and other care workers who can become involved in the care of one person.

It may be that in the future the current tendency toward specialization will become blurred in the interests of promoting teamwork. Whatever the future may bring the vision of integrated collaborative care must remain or primary care will become pre-occupied with the problems themselves at the expense of their solution.

References

1 Castledine G (1996) Cutting across traditional specialist community nursing boundaries. *Br J Comm Health Nursing* **1**(1):57–8.
2 Twinn S (1996) Introduction – nursing for community health: changing professional issues, in *Community Health Care Nursing: principles for practice* (eds Twinn S, Roberts B and Andrews S). Butterworth Heinemann, Oxford.
3 Reid T and David A (1994) Primary care nursing. Community Nursing Practice management and teamwork. *Nursing Times* **21**:42–5.
4 Pietroni P (1992) Beyond the boundaries: relationship between general practice and complementary medicine. *BMJ* **305**:564–6.
5 Jones D (1996) Epidemiology II: care of older people in community health, in *Community Health Nursing: frameworks for practice* (eds Gastrell P and Edwards J). Baillière Tindall, London.
6 NHSME Value for Money Unit (1992) *The Nursing Skill Mix in the District Nursing Service.* HMSO, London.
7 Waine C (1992) The primary care team [editorial]. *Br J Gen Pract* **42**:498–9.
8 Baldock J and Ungerson C (1994) *Becoming consumers of Community Care: households within the mixed economy of welfare.* Joseph Rowntree Foundation, York.
9 Beales D and Saffin K (1995) *Experiences of care following hip fracture.* Unpublished research report. Unit of Epidemiology, University of Oxford.
10 Parker G and Beales D (1993) Provision to reflect real needs. *Professional Nurse* **Sept**:820–4.

Further reading

Gastrell P and Edwards J (eds) (1996) *Community Health Nursing. frameworks for practice.* Baillière Tindall, London.
Pritchard P and Pritchard J (1993) *Developing Teamwork in Primary Health Care: a practical workbook. Practical Guides for General Practice 15.* Oxford Medical Publications, Oxford.
SSI/DoH/NISW (1993) *Empowerment, Assessment, Care Management and the Skilled Worker.* HMSO, London.

Acknowledgement

I would like to thank Colin Hughes CPN for his help in preparing the section on community psychiatric nursing.

CHAPTER 11

Institutional care of older people in the community

Clive Bowman

In the wake of the 1990 NHS reforms the continuing care provision for elderly people has changed beyond recognition. Previously, long-term care had been typically provided by the NHS in old Victorian infirmaries and similar outmoded facilities. The weakness of the poor physical characteristics of traditional NHS accommodation deflected attention from the important contribution of established professional coordination and a wide-ranging nursing and paramedical support. In this setting for long-term care much wisdom and good practice had been established via the cycle of inadequacy – scandal – standard setting. Changes in policy since then have meant that inadequacy is difficult to establish without a coherent regulatory framework to oversee standards in the greatly increased range of provider settings.

Institutional care in the community is now provided by many independent or corporate residential and nursing homes. Those requiring state support are means assessed by social service officers and the cost is met by local authorities. In 1996, health authorities became obliged to define criteria for NHS continuing care criteria on health grounds. There still are no national guidelines for establishing who requires continuing hospital care, residential or nursing care. Only small numbers of physically or mentally disabled people are supported directly by health authorities in continuing care establishments and this creates tension between the health authority and social service budgets. Fees paid by local authorities are £100 a week less when someone is placed in residential accommodation and this may lead to inappropriate placement for those with the need for continuing nursing care.

Inadequacy of placement or appropriate care will be difficult to establish in the present circumstances as care has been isolated from the traditional statutory monitoring instruments, such as the health advisory service. The new markets of health and care have encouraged simplistic purchasing with dubious targets, quality assurance schemes and an increasingly elusive 'buck stops here' responsibility for the chronically sick in long-term nursing care.

Presently, there are some 170 000 nursing home beds in England and Wales. The routine medical supervision of these patients poses an increasing challenge to the already stretched resources of primary care. In many retirement areas of the UK a general practitioner (GP) with an average list of 2000 patients may have a practice population containing 29% over 65 years and around 100 people in institutional care scattered over several homes. In such circumstances the demands on GPs are indeed onerous and it is not surprising that in the debate over core and non-core service the General Medical Services Committee of the British Medical Association has proposed exclusion of those with severe physical care needs from core service provision by GPs.

Where care is provided in nursing homes it usually offers advantages over old condemned facilities, particularly with regard to environment.

Diverse standards for accommodation, staffing and regimens have been developed, however, and promoted typically without widespread evaluation. The shift to long-term care in nursing homes represents a transformation from multi-disciplinary team care for the individual in typically hostile institutions, to a domesticated care environment with an isolation or even divorce from health services care and support. The cornerstone of care in this field is the establishment and management of patient needs with an appropriate level and skill-mix of staff following an initial streaming assessment. Standards need to be set with an effective registration and inspection service. Care needs to be flexible enough to allow appropriate and rapid response to sudden care need changes and access to aids and appliances for basic care needs, such as transferring and bathing and pressure care. This must also be cost-effective. Processes that seem to require medical involvement include:

- initial assessment
- care planning
- systematized care
- routine surveillance
- risk management
- quality assurance.

These facets are considered below using case studies.

Assessment

The cost of long-term care justifies the need for a properly considered assessment. Patients need to have their medical state and their present and future care needs identified and defined. They can then be streamed into appropriate care, for example, residential, nursing, elderly mentally infirm (EMI), residential or nursing care. At this point, assessment has only directed the patient into a form of care. After admission, a structured assessment then defines and guides care planning. It is imperative that professional nurse care staff have adequate medical information on which to build their care package. The consequences of expediency are illustrated in the following case study.

Case study

A normally independent 77-year-old widow was admitted to hospital following a fall in which a head injury led to transient loss of consciousness. She remained confused over several weeks in hospital. She was diagnosed as suffering from epilepsy and parkinsonism for which treatments were commenced. Slow progress led after three weeks to her friends being advised that discharge to a nursing home, for long-term care, was necessary. Her home was subsequently sold.

Some months later she recovered and spent much time walking the streets to 'escape' the nursing home. Subsequently, she moved to a residential home where she remains well – over ten years on from the initial fall. She can now clearly recall her fall being due to a trip on a loose stair carpet. There is no evidence of parkinsonism or epilepsy. It is clear that a head injury led to a concussed state misinterpreted by the responsible hospital team and that this assessment was accepted without question by her GP.

The importance of an unhurried interview with families and carers cannot be overemphasized, particularly in the presence of cognitive impairment, to obtain an appreciation of the issues in each case. Rehabilitation of the elderly man with advanced prostatic carcinoma and paraplegia related to disease spread will have a very different set of goals from the patient with a fractured neck of femur following an isolated fall. Communication and enquiry are often potentially fraught with carers, family and friends often charged with frustration, anger, disappointment, unrealistic expectations and exhaustion. In difficult circumstances formulations for action must not be rushed into. When decisions are made in an unhurried way practical policy underpinned by common sense is likely to command a wide consensus of support. Similarly, it is helpful for all concerned to be aware of the processes and time required for adequate assessment.

Multidimensional assessment tools of varying sophistication are available. A consistency in application is important with the need to be able to communicate to a variety of agencies in a recognized, intelligible language. Well-validated assessment scales are important in the measurement of mental state and physical function. The Abbreviated Mental Test and the Barthel Activities of Daily Living assessment (ADL) have been endorsed by the Royal College of Physicians and the British Geriatrics Society. These are easily applied and if accompanied by a descriptive narrative, give a reliable picture of a patient's clinical state. Sequential assessments of ADL are useful in evaluating rehabilitative progress.

Planned admission to a residential or nursing home should be accompanied by a clear medical, mental, functional and social assessment for establishing a base-line that guides care planning and facilitating subsequent review. Primary care teams can also apply this information to define and use an objective index of functional state as a measure of health status change.

Care planning

Good preparation and multi-disciplinary casework make care management successful. Particular difficulties may arise with cognitive impairment where there may be a need for proxy decision-making by family and/or legal appointees. In all circumstances, the multi-disciplinary consensus must be communicated clearly and consistently. When extended families (often with widely differing aspirations) are given inconsistent advice from hospital staff this leads to confusion and detracts from the needs of the patient.

The appropriate form of community institutional setting is important. In general, a residential home should offer the level of care that could be expected to be provided by an able family. Nursing-home care should be provided for those needing more skilled and specialized nursing care. The lack of precision in definition allows both flexibility and exposes individuals to risk. An ambulant demented person may well be suited to specialist residential care for the EMI. More challenging behaviour, in particular aggressive tendencies and/or major continence problems, make a nursing EMI home or unit more suitable. Conversely, a heavily physically dependent person with major cognitive impairment may be more appropriately managed in a frail elderly unit. The potential for this flexibility to encourage the cheapest care solution to be accepted as adequate produces many pressures in an environment of limited resources. Residential/nursing care borderline cases, where progressive decline in health status can be anticipated, should be clearly communicated so that care with the ability to adapt to increasing need is given proper consideration.

Patients assessed as fit for residential care may have a dependence masked by the level of care and support being received, for example, whilst in hospital care.

Determining the optimal solution for an individual must involve not only the proximity of a home to an individual's roots but also be mindful of their ethnic origin, social class, choice, personality and idiosyncrasies. Achieving the ideal match of these variables in the context of often limited options is clearly difficult and the realistic 'best fit' compromise should be offered. A review can then be made later.

Providing accurate and adequate information is a major responsibility for hospital or primary care teams involved in the referral and transfer of patients to community institutional care. Clear communication is essential to allow new medical advocates to be able to make reasonable management decisions, as shown in the case study below.

Case study

An 85-year-old man discharged from an acute hospital bed with terminal cardiorespiratory disease to a private nursing home was severely distressed on admission. Medical documentation had been put in the post to the newly responsible GP who was asked to review the patient at the nursing home shortly after the patient's admission. Unfamiliar with the patient's clinical condition the GP referred the patient back to hospital. In the Accident & Emergency department the patient was re-examined by the resident medical officer, familiar with the patient's status and discharged back to the nursing home. The patient died shortly after.

Care planning by nursing staff is dependent on a clear understanding of a medical state so that reasonable care objectives and prognoses can be established. Attending doctors need adequate information to understand the medical status of the patient as well as a clear picture of functional status to enable the significance of change to be understood.

The presence of properly constructed advance directives or living wills should be determined and recorded. Though difficult, it is important, if a patient has the cognitive and communication abilities, to enquire about preferences. If proper directives have been made their presence must be clearly stated on the medical summary and in nursing records. A legally empowered advocate should be clearly recorded together with his or her status, e.g. activated enduring power of attorney and their responsibilities respected.

Systematized care

The workload generated for primary care teams by a large nursing home causes much consternation. Problems are assured if careful operational planning is not undertaken! The adoption of a reactive stance will neither contain the workload nor serve the often complex clinical needs of patients. A well organized approach by the primary care team is vital to provide good standards of care. Also a programmed approach defines the needs and solutions which in turn anticipates problems, reduces emergency work and improves communication, confidence and care by the primary care and nursing home teams.

Case study

A large nursing home opened in the catchment of a group practice, much to the consternation of the six partners who found themselves responsible for 60 frail elderly residents who had been admitted from hospital beds. Initially, the partners adopted a reactive approach which meant increased emergency calls, discontinuity of care and a frustration among care staff with whom relationships became increasingly fraught. A review highlighted the need for an operational policy that recognized the needs of patients, the care staff and the real constraints on primary care resources. The practice contained two partners who had experienced geriatric medicine in training and the 60 patients were divided between these partners who each made a weekly planned visit to the home. Each designated partner agreed to review five patients per visit which meant each patient was seen together with a senior nurse every two months. The senior nurse listed non-urgent problems and issues for attention in residents not being formally reviewed and a diary of actions such as routine blood testing was established. Admissions to the nursing home were

planned to be shortly before a scheduled visit which aided co-operation. A major reduction in emergency calls followed and the practice and nursing home care staff developed a good working practice based on shared-care values and mutual confidence. The practice found that it could provide terminal care and respite care to its patients within the home having developed good working practices with local social workers maintaining continuity of care.

A system of regular patient review affords a means to establish patterns of care that not only meet patients' immediate needs but allow a predictability of response to issues. Time spent on specific components of an individual's medical state will generate a unique set of clinical guidelines which, if properly applied, will lead to appropriate care and use medical time effectively as well as allowing nurses to develop appropriate care plans.

Routine surveillance

The routine surveillance of dependent long-term care patients is not adequately covered by the 'over-75' screening programme. Dentures, hearing aids, appliances and aids generally need to be reviewed; many of these may be monitored by nursing staff but medical referral may be required for repair or reassessment. For example, most patients with hearing impairment are issued with 'behind the ear' hearing aids. Commonly nursing-home patients lack the manipulative skills to use these and as a consequence may become increasingly isolated, leading to a perception of deteriorating mental function. A simple body-worn aid with an earpiece may, however, be manageable and bring significant benefits to the individual. It is also salutary to observe how well-fitting, comfortable footwear can enhance independence!

Formal reviews of medication are essential, therapeutic areas that cause frequent difficulties are psychotropics and diuretics. Diuretic therapy for cardiac failure is seldom reviewed. Psychotropic drugs are commonly prescribed as a response to distressed and distressing behaviour which may represent a phase of dementing illness or simply a reaction to the unfamiliarity of a new environment. If the appropriateness of initiation of psychotropic drugs is a complex issue, ongoing prescribing is almost certainly one of the most uncertain areas of therapeutics.

Weight measurements can provide a useful objective indicator and a sensitive trigger for the review of a wide range of care issues, providing they are seen in context of a clinical situation. The patient with cardiac cachexia may be expected to exhibit a steady weight loss. However, the patient with an impaired ability to swallow following stroke may be losing weight due to swallowing difficulties, poor food preparation or even inadequate nursing assistance with feeding.

Risk management

Infection control is of great importance in hospitals where multiple resistant organisms pose major clinical risks. Nursing homes, for infection-control purposes, exhibit many similarities to acute hospitals. The residents are often immuno-compromised through chronic disease and exposed to risk by, for example, indwelling catheters. Frequent, repeated infection and multiple courses of antibiotics encourage nosocomial infections. Close co-operation with microbiology departments and agreed antibiotic policies are clearly desirable.

Annual influenza immunization is an important component of risk management and should be planned for all elderly in institutional care.

Falls are common in institutional patients with impaired mobility and repeated falls should trigger a formal case review to understand and minimize risk factors, which may range from the disarmingly simple, to the revision of complex anti-parkinsonian therapy and the detection and management of postural hypotension.

Pressure area management if actively practised clearly offers the prospect of pressure-sore avoidance. Nursing staff routinely assess pressure-sore formation risk using typically the Waterlow or Norton scales. Warnings should be acted on. A patient with Parkinson's disease whose risk suddenly rises due to an intercurrent infection, should be managed aggressively with large air-cell pressure-relieving mattresses. This example also highlights the need for risk assessment to be a dynamic process, not one just undertaken on admission.

Quality assurance

The classical Donabedian approach considering structure, process and outcome is as relevant to long-term care patients as any other patient groups. The physical environment of institutional care in the community has improved as a result of good inspection mechanisms for residential care homes by the local authority and for nursing homes by the health authority. This review system does not take into account the appropriateness of the care provided for people of widely differing dependency needs, and in assessing the process of care, registration teams have a limited brief. They have little ability within their mandate and resources to undertake individual case-care quality assurance. Individual residents will certainly want the best outcome of care possible. Outcome expectations may range from maximization of autonomy and life quality in the face of a handicap, in effect a rehabilitative stance, to palliative care for a terminal malignancy. With this spectrum of activity, a clear perception of quality is difficult. Considering the cost of long-term care this situation is unacceptable. Outcome assessment starts with the naive questions 'Was, or is, it the right thing to do and was, or is, it done correctly'? Clinical audit becomes the tool whereby outcome is assessed after agreeing acceptable standards.

Future possibilities

There is an increasing body of opinion seeking the establishment of a single registration of community care homes. However, within the present distinction between residential and nursing homes there is likely to be a greater sophistication of skill-mix and supportive infrastructure. In simple terms it is probable that generally frail elderly people in residential care with modest demands on health services will remain the responsibility of primary care. More dependent nursing cases will require, as at present professional nurse-led care, but this should be underpinned by specific case management.

The minimum data set (MDS) – resident assessment protocols (RAPs) – established as a statutory process in the US, and spreading widely, offers a pragmatic way forward for developing outcomes based on long-term care. Of particular importance, the assessment protocols offer a means for primary and secondary care to provide structured managed care across a number of health issues in an accountable manner. It is probable that the development of national standards will identify a highly dependent; but small cadre of individuals whose needs would be best met by specialist-led long-term care in a health authority facility, even though this may be a nursing home unit.

The future therefore for the overburdened and unsupported GP could be resolved through a facilitation of care of nursing home patients supported by item-of-service payments and a removal of the most dependent care consumers to specialist-led care.

For mental impairment a similar and parallel set of arrangements integrating primary and secondary care is needed; with extreme impairment accompanied by challenging behaviour being more accountably the responsibility of secondary care.

Cost pressures imposed on long-term care are inevitably going to lead to economies of scale. Homes will become larger. This will have the effect of concentrating the people with complex health needs rather than disseminating them in the community. It will also concentrate skilled nursing staff.

The endangered skills and traditions of geriatric medicine are likely to become re-established but in the community where they will contribute to a seamless care approach to the frail elderly.

National standards and a systematic approach to inspection are overdue. For example, in school education, where a National Curriculum monitored and developed through a structured inspection service, has led to standard setting, understanding and progress.

Key points

Individuals in long-term care should receive individualized, multi-disciplinary assessments from which care plans and managed medical care and surveillance can be developed.

- Assessment is a continuous process not a rite of passage on admission

- Case management requires careful documentation, consideration and good communication

- Long-term care leadership in multi-disciplinary teams is earned not bestowed

- Long-term care management is most obvious when it is most deficient

CHAPTER 12

Disability and rehabilitation for older people

Sean Brotheridge and John Young

One of the founders of geriatric medicine, Joseph Sheldon (1893–1972), described by some as the 'father of community geriatric care', was one of the first investigators to highlight the problems of older people living at home, especially those of poor mobility, falls and impaired vision and hearing. He recognized that most disabled elderly people wish to remain at home and this could only be achieved by increasing community support and providing support for caring families. Many of Sheldon's themes remain pivotal in the management of contemporary older disabled people living at home.

Impairment, disability and handicap

Few elderly people suffer from a single disease but instead have several chronic degenerative processes, a fact which is reflected in the increase in impairment, disability and handicap with advancing years.

It is estimated that 4.3 million older people (over 60 years of age) are disabled in the UK, representing 70% of all disabled people or nearly 50% of all elderly people. The vast majority of older disabled people live in their own homes, with impaired mobility as the most frequent disability category (see Box 12.1).

According to the World Health Organisation's 'International Classification of Impairments, Disabilities and Handicap' (1980), any illness can be considered at the levels of pathology, impairment, disability and handicap.

Impairment: Any loss or abnormality of psychological, physiological or anatomical structure or function.

Disability: Any restriction or lack of ability (resulting from an impairment) to perform an activity in a manner or within a range considered normal.

Box 12.1: Frequency of disability types in over 75-year-olds living at home

Mobility	82%
Hearing	55%
Personal care	46%
Vision	40%
Dexterity	33%
Continence	21%
Communication	20%

Box 12.2: Much apparent 'disability' is located outwith the person

> Consider an elderly lady who has lumbar spondylosis (pathology) resulting in a stiff, poorly mobile spine (impairment) such that she cannot bend down to plug in an electrical appliance (disability) and is therefore unable to do her ironing (handicap). Simply raising her electric socket to mid-thigh height abolishes the handicap even though the pathology, impairment and disability are unchanged.

Handicap: A disadvantage for a given individual, resulting from an impairment or disability, that limits or prevents their fulfilment of a role that would be normal for that individual.

This classification framework is a very useful systematic model within which to consider the rehabilitation process. It prompts the need to uncover a cause (pathology or impairment) for the disability when a person presents with, for example, a mobility problem; whilst also prompting examination of the consequences of the disease in functional terms (disability) and in relation to the lifestyle and environment of the individual patient (handicap). Thus a balanced approach is achieved between disease modification (usually drugs) and maximizing independence (physical treatments, aids and adaptations). It reinforces the rehabilitationist's obsession with environment modification, as much 'disability' is located outwith the person in environments constructed for able-bodied people (see Box 12.2).

Measurement of impairment

Measurement of impairment relies on clinical examination aided by bedside tests and/or standardized assessments. Some examples are given below:

- vision   Snellen chart
- hearing   whispering into ear
- joints   range of motion measurement
- cognition   Abbreviated Mental Test Score
- speech   Frenchay Aphasia Screening Test
- gait   timed 5-metre walk
- breathing   peak expiratory flow rate

Measurement of disability

In the field of rehabilitation research numerous scales have been developed to quantify aspects of disability. Few have found routine clinical applications. Perhaps the most widely used measure in both hospitals and the community is the Barthel Index score (see Figure 12.1). It assesses levels of independence or dependence for ten activities of daily living (ADL) with a score range of 0 (dependent) to 20 (independent). This score is quick and easy to use, has been carefully researched and can aid both systematic disability assessment and also show rehabilitation progress if repeated at intervals. The main disadvantages of the Barthel Index are that the steps on the scale are fairly large – it is therefore not very sensitive to change; and that, especially for disabled people living at home, there is a marked 'ceiling' effect in as much as patients can score a maximum of 20 points and be 'independent' but still have daily living restrictions. Nevertheless, the Barthel Index provides a valuable tool to assess disabled elderly people and its routine use has much to commend it.

Some workers have extended the range of the Barthel Index to include important other daily living tasks such as housework, shopping and trips. These scales are referred to as 'extended' or 'instrumental ADL scales'. Examples include the Nottingham Extended ADL Scale and the Frenchay Activities Index: both designed for use with stroke patients.

Disease-specific disability scales have been developed for some conditions such as arthritis, Parkinson's disease and multiple sclerosis and could be considered for use in specialized clinics.

Measuring handicap

This is an active area of current research but no routine approach to the documentation of handicap has yet been developed. However, considerable insight into handicap can be gained by careful clinical observation but usually only

Surname:
First Names:
Unit No:
Date: Ward:

Task	Usual	Current	Week 1	Week 2	Week 3	Week 4	Disch	Scoring Criteria
Dressing								2 = Independent - ties shoes, copes with zips etc. 1 = Needs help but does half in a reasonable time 0 = Dependent
Feeding								2 = Independent - reasonable speed 1 = Needs help - cutting food 0 = Unable
Grooming								1 = Face/Hair/Teeth/Shaves all on own 0 = Dependent
Toilet								2 = Independent 1 = Needs help 0 = Unable
Bathing								1 = Independent 0 = Dependent
Bed/Chair Transfers								3 = Totally independent 2 = Minimal help needed 1 = Heavily dependent 0 = Unable
Ambulation								3 = Independent or - may use an aid 2 = With help of one person 1 = Wheelchair, but independent 0 = Immobile
Stairs								2 = Independent 1 = Needs help 0 = Unable
Bladder								2 = No accidents, manages catheter if *in situ* 1 = Occasional accidents/ needs help with catheter if *in situ* 0 = Incontinent
Bowels								2 = No accidents 1 = Occasional accidents/ needs help with enemas etc. 0 = Incontinent
Total								

Figure 12.1 Barthel Index score

when the disabled older person is assessed in the context of their own home.

Assessment of older people with disability

There are three processes in the management of older people with disabilities:

1 a sound assessment and analysis of problems

2 intervention to reduce impairment, disability and handicap

3 an evaluation of the effectiveness of these interventions.

The first step is an initial assessment. This must be accurate and relevant to an individual's needs so that any future interventions are meaningful. In the community setting most people with complex disability will currently receive a 'comprehensive assessment'. This process has been stimulated by the 1990 Community Care Act. It involves the completion of a complex document by several health care professionals which draws together aspects of health and social care requirements; from nursing care and mobility, to dressing ability, toileting and feeding. The process and imple- mentation is coordinated by a social worker.

Each professional discipline will have been trained within a specific system for disability assessment. However, it is important to recognize that there is no simple general 'formula' or check-list system which can be universally ap- plied in disability assessment. Although there are several general themes, particularly mobility re- striction and carer support, it is the individuality of each patient that must be explored. A 'relaxed–attention' observation style is therefore appropriate. Relaxed in the sense of being un- focused and aware of both verbal and non-verbal messages; taking note of the person's surround- ings; their interaction with them; but attentive so that clues are not missed but can be picked up on in later questioning. A useful general approach is shown in Box 12.3, based upon three sequential steps.

Box 12.3: Disability assessment steps

Step 1
Divergent phase to identify problems using open questions and to encourage patients/carers to give their own accounts.

Step 2
Convergent phase with focused questions to define and refine diagnosis, disability and handicap (see Box 12.4).

Step 3
A further divergent phase to ensure comprehensiveness using techniques such as:
● Are there any other problems not yet explored?
● Completing the Barthel Index as a check-list to cover systematically important areas of disability such as incontinence, toilet transfers, which may have been overlooked.
● Asking the care-giver(s) to recount a typical 24 hour care-giver day.

The role of rehabilitation

In 1958 the World Health Organisation stated that:

> medical rehabilitation has the fundamental objective not only of restoring the disabled person to his or her previous condition, but also of developing the person to the maximum extent of their physical and mental functions.

Older people with chronic disease cannot always be returned to their previous condition. Some- times the underlying disease is progressive (e.g. chronic heart failure, motor neurone disease). Sometimes the disease leaves irreparable damage (e.g. stroke, trauma). Therefore a more appropriate concept for rehabilitation in older people is to consider it as a 'complex set of processes usually involving several professional disciplines and aimed at improving the quality of life of older people facing daily living difficulties.' (Figure 12.2.)

It is important to recognize that rehabilitation is not a short 'quick-fix' process. An adequate time frame is required – usually weeks and

Box 12.4: Disability assessment

Personal features	
Gait	– Always ask patient to walk, and
	– check aids
Feet and shoes	– Check
Vision and spectacles	– Check
Hearing and aids	– Check
Medication	– Gather them up and check dates
Home features	
Heating	– Check if person can turn fire on/off
Lighting	– Advise high wattage in corridors and stairways
Food	– Check fridge and cupboard
Stairs	– Extra rail needed?
Bathroom	– Bath aids needed?
Toilet	– Rails or raised seat needed?
Mobility obstacles	– Furniture, steps, loose carpeting etc.
Outside home	
Access	– Step to doorways?
Neighbours	– May be part of caring network
Shops/bank etc.	– Near or far?

months. Moreover, patients may move between active rehabilitation – where the expectation is on improving functional ability; and maintenance rehabilitation – where the expectation is prevention of deterioration. Both involve the same overall approach (Figure 12.2) and both are important if disabled older people are to remain in their own homes.

Evidence for the effectiveness of community (home) rehabilitation has accumulated slowly. For example, domiciliary occupational therapy advice, treatment and aids provision caused a significant improvement in daily living skills for a group of elderly people with rheumatoid arthritis. Home physiotherapy has improved independence for patients with stroke, Parkinson's disease and knee arthritis. Also, a course of three domiciliary physiotherapy sessions has been shown to improve mobility and balance in elderly people following a fall. 'Hospital-at-home' schemes (essentially augmented home-nursing care services) have been developed in some areas and it has then been possible to transfer the rehabilitation of selected patients with a fractured neck of femur from the hospital setting to the home.

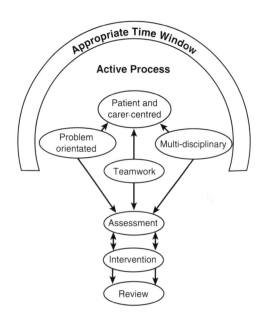

Figure 12.2 Core concepts of rehabilitation

The multi-disciplinary team

Underpinning the process of rehabilitation, either in the hospital or within the community, is the notion of the multi-disciplinary team. The members of this team may vary from setting to setting, and patient to patient. But in the community it generally comprises the general practitioner (GP), district nurse, social worker, home-care team manager, community physiotherapist and community occupational therapist. The social worker has a special coordinating role in relation to the Community Care Act and has budgetary control for the social services' contribution to care arrangements. It should be noted that an essential aspect of community rehabilitation, especially for older disabled people living alone at home, is provision of general supportive care. Therefore, involvement of the home care team and community nursing is essential and if either of these is deficient the rehabilitation interventions may fail.

In an ideal team, the members share a common purpose which binds them together and guides their actions. Each member of the team should have a clear understanding of their own roles, appreciate and understand the contributions of other professions in the team and recognize common interest and skills. The effectiveness of this team is related to its ability to carry out its work and to manage itself as an inter-dependent group of people.

Working in the community requires skills and experience beyond those necessary in the closed, supportive environment of a hospital ward. It is harder to support, supervise, coordinate and train when staff are working in isolation, or in small teams away from a central base. One of the main instruments of communication that can maintain a community rehabilitation team is the telephone and this is increasingly being supplemented by e-mail. Each member of the team generally observes an 'office session', usually early in the morning, when it is mutually understood that members will be available for telephone contact at their base. This understanding gives the opportunity for team members to exchange views, make referrals and generally maintain the rapport required to ensure that the processes of rehabilitation occur effectively.

Community physiotherapists

Community physiotherapists are mostly employed by health service trusts but social services may employ some physiotherapists for special projects and services, most commonly to provide assessment and treatment for disabled elderly people in institutional care. Increasingly, fund-holding general practices will employ physiotherapists directly as part of their primary care team.

The physiotherapist is concerned with physical treatments and advice to improve movement – especially walking – but also standing up, sitting up from a bed, transferring between chair and commode, and managing stairs and steps safely. Part of their work involves assessment and provision of correct walking aids and referrals for wheelchairs. They can also help to improve upper-limb and hand-function affected, for example, by arthritis or stroke.

Community occupational therapists

Occupational therapists may work for health trusts or social services. The role and duties of the occupational therapist vary between these two agencies. Social service occupational therapists usually hold an equipment and adaptations budget with which they provide small aids (such as bathing aids, kitchen aids) or home adaptations (such as ramps to front door, between-floor lifts, stair-lifts). They are often (unfairly) criticized because of the long delays which ensue whilst disabled people wait for their alterations. It is simply that their budget allocation is insufficient to cope with the demands made upon it.

The health trust occupational therapists also assess need for equipment and adaptations (usually referring on the patient's requirements to colleague occupational therapists in the social services) and undertake treatment sessions to help, for example, improve independence in kitchen work, dressing and bathing. Their role overlaps with the community physiotherapist in teaching carers transfer techniques or use of equipment, such as raised toilet seats and hoists.

Rehabilitation goals

The process of setting goals is central to the management of the older person with disabilities and their rehabilitation. These goals should be precise statements, agreed by patients, carers and the multi-disciplinary team so that their achievement is unambiguous. As well as being realistic to the patient, they should be well communicated to all involved, and documented. Failure to achieve a goal does not necessarily mean that a particular rehabilitation intervention has failed – there are other possible reasons:

- an inaccurate initial assessment was made

- unrealistic goals were set

- the intervention was inappropriate

- insufficient time was given for the achievement of the goal.

It is important to remember that rehabilitation progress may be slowed by undiagnosed medical problems (such as anaemia, cardiac failure), or occult depression, occult dementia and communication problems (deafness or poor eyesight).

Rehabilitation services in the community

Day hospitals

Community rehabilitation does not necessarily have to occur within the disabled person's home. A well-established service for older people in this country is the day hospital. Day hospitals, developed during a period when community care was rudimentary, aimed to provide comprehensive nursing, medical and rehabilitative care for old people as an alternative to hospital admission. Many day hospitals are now altering their role to provide a more flexible range of community-based services, such as home physiotherapy, occupational therapy and speech therapy in close liaison with local social services. The therapists either treat people within their own home, or provide transport to bring the patients to the day-hospital base, perhaps just for an hour or so rather than the four to six hour day which was traditional day-hospital practice.

Day hospitals are also staffed by medical practitioners: usually GPs who have developed a special interest in care of older people. They are generally employed for a two to four hour session under the guidance of a consultant geriatrician who will hold clinics and case conferences at weekly intervals, or more frequently.

This health care environment therefore provides an ideal base for an integrated multi-disciplinary assessment of disabled older people, perhaps more attuned to their rehabilitation in the community, and in contrast to a potentially disjointed hospital outpatient service with separate visits to the doctor, various therapists and social services staff.

Home- or centre-based rehabilitation

Advantages of home care:

- no uncomfortable travel by the patient

- greater flexibility of treatment provision

- greater opportunity for carer involvement

- greater likelihood of addressing handicap rather than the disability

- more integrated programme of care

- care and follow up more frequently by the same care worker

- relief for the carer.

Disadvantages of home care:

- patient is denied the social dimension of day-hospital visit

- home environment may be too cluttered and cramped which impedes the rehabilitation process

- there might be a need for special equipment which the therapist could not carry with them.

All these factors need to be taken into account in deciding which site is preferable in each individual case.

Home discharge

Rehabilitation services in the community should closely complement the achievements of hospital rehabilitation. It has been recognized that sometimes the hospital staff do not see beyond the

Box 12.5: Sources of aids and equipment

Walking aids	– physiotherapy service
Kitchen/bath and toilet aids	– social service or health trust occupational therapists
Pendant alarm	– social services office
Wheelchairs	– wheelchair service
Home adaptations	– social services occupational therapists
Special mattresses } Commodes	– home loans service (via community nurses)

patient's discharge. Methods of sustaining the rehabilitation process and preventing dissipation of functional improvements need to be considered. For example, some patients with a hemiplegic stroke continue to make slow functional recovery for many months after the initial three-month rapid recovery phase, and many disabled elderly people deteriorate functionally when they leave a closely supportive hospital ward environment. Hospital discharge should therefore provide an opportunity for smooth transition to the community rehabilitation team and to draw on its knowledge and experience in how to maintain functional ability and reduce handicap. A valuable opportunity for handover is during a predischarge home assessment visit. Here the patient is taken home for an hour or so by the hospital rehabilitation staff to identify areas of concern and plan appropriate support services and equipment needed.

Aids for daily living

The contribution of daily living aids in reducing handicap for older disabled people cannot be stressed strongly enough. Currently, however, the provision of aids can be a complex process and one which varies from area to area. Certain general statements apply, but those involved with the care of disabled people need to apply themselves and learn their local procedures for referral. It is clear that effective provision of aids can be a major barrier to successful rehabilitation. It can also highlight the difficulty in communication between hospital wards and the community. Unfortunately, many aids and pieces of equipment go unused by the patient. Careful selection, discussion with the patient and training

in the use of the aid or equipment will reduce this non-use.

Examples include wheelchairs which can be obtained from designated wheelchair centres. However their use may depend upon a ramp to the patient's home, organized by social services, generally after an appreciable delay. Kitchen and dressing aids are available after assessment by social services occupational therapists, whilst bathing and toilet aids are provided from the social services area offices (see Box 12.5). The provision process would be improved by a single centre from which all aids could be obtained after appropriate assessment. Such a centre could conceivably also be the base for the local community rehabilitation team and a coordinating centre for information services to help and support disabled older people and their carers.

Conclusion

The potential advantages of community care, as envisaged within the 1990 Community Care Act, include greater autonomy and choice for both young and old disabled people, care provision which is tailored to individual need and a flexible use of public, private and voluntary services. In many areas these aspirations have been slow to realize. The opportunity for community-based rehabilitation relies heavily on GPs and their primary care teams taking the initiative. It is important that rehabilitation referral routes are well known and easy to contact. Conversely, rehabilitation staff need to be visible and to build bridges to the primary health care team.

Rehabilitation concepts are being steadily developed but sometimes the expertise being applied within hospital centres does not reach the population with the greatest need, i.e. older disabled people living at home. Variations in context and quality of community rehabilitation across the UK need to be addressed so that good services are available to all people, no matter where they live. Moves towards shortening hospital stay by domiciliary rehabilitation using, for example, 'hospital-at-home' schemes remain attractive but need continuing careful evaluation to confirm that they achieve their clinical objectives and are cost-effective.

More generally, the advances to improve understanding and communication between hospital and community rehabilitation staff need continued attention.

Further reading

Andrews K (1991) *Rehabilitation of the older adult*. Edward Arnold, London.

Donaldson RJ and Donaldson LJ (1987) *Essential Community Medicine*. MTP Press. Chapters 5 and 8.

Mulley G (1989) *Everyday Aids and Appliances*. BMJ Publishing, London.

Owens P, Carrier J and Horder J (1995) *Interprofessional Issues in Community and Primary Health Care*. Macmillan Press, London.

Sheldon JH (1948) *The Social Medicine of Old Age*. Oxford University Press, London.

DoH (1992) *The Health of Elderly People: An epidemiological overview*. HMSO, London.

Wade DT (1992) Stroke rehabilitation, in *The Oxford Textbook of Geriatric Medicine* (eds Grimley Evans J, Franklin Williams T), Oxford Medical Publications, Oxford.

CHAPTER 13

Special services for older people

David Lubel

This chapter considers the wide range of services available to older people and their carers in the community. Few evolved specifically for the use of the older person yet these services form the cornerstone of community care of older people.

The origins of community care

The concept of community care did not flourish in Victorian Britain, particularly with the passing of the 1834 amendment to the 1601 Poor Relief Act. This virtually eliminated non-institutional assistance to the needy by denying relief to those who refused to enter 'workhouses'. By the turn of the century, public opinion was changing and it was considered unfair to group the elderly and infirm with the 'unworthy' poor. Institutional care was becoming discredited and provision of assistance and care at home was considered a cheaper option. With the creation of the National Health Service (NHS) in 1948 the aim was to provide a network of care for the whole population 'from the cradle to the grave', the state being seen as 'the universal provider'. The need for change was becoming apparent by the 1980s. The inexorable rise in numbers of elderly people in the population seemed to be placing ever increasing demands on the nation's finances. This was exemplified by the cost to the state of funding residential and nursing care, which increased a hundred-fold during the 1980s, reaching £1000 million a year by 1990. The government believed that insufficient support in the community was forcing people into institutional care – the so-called 'perverse incentive' – and at the same time the NHS was also saving money by cutting long-stay provision and leaving people with no alternative. In 1986 Sir Roy Griffiths was asked to review the way in which public funds were being used to support community care policy. Based on the findings of the Griffiths Report, the government introduced the 1990 NHS and Community Care Act. As a result of this legislation social services departments (SSDs) ceased to be mere suppliers of services, and instead assumed the lead role in assessing social care needs and commissioning services. The Act had six key objectives which are outlined in Box 13.1.

The primary objective was to reduce spending on the social services by a process of rationalization and rationing.

Who provides community care?

Informal carers

The major burden of care for the frail elderly lies with informal unpaid carers: relatives, friends and neighbours and the hidden costs are considered greatly to exceed public and private spending. The importance of informal carers and their specific needs was recognized by the Carers (Recognition and Services) Act 1995 (in force from 1 April 1996). For the first time, carers have been given the right to an assessment of their own ability to perform the caring task.

Box 13.1: Key objectives of the NHS and Community Care Act 1990

- To promote the development of domiciliary, day care and respite care services to enable people to live in their own homes

- To ensure that proper assessment of need and good care management are cornerstones

- To ensure that service providers make practical support for carers a high priority

- To clarify the responsibilities of agencies and make them responsible

- To promote the development of a flourishing, independent sector alongside good quality public services and for SSDs to become enabling agencies making best use of private and voluntary providers

- To secure better value for taxpayers' money by introducing a new funding structure for social care

Formal care-providers

The main formal providers of community care services are outlined in Box 13.2. A consequence of the NHS and Community Care Act has been to improve collaboration between SSDs and health services and increase public spending within the private and voluntary sectors. The intention has been to create a 'mixed economy of care' and to

Box 13.2: Major providers of community care services for older people

- Local authority social services departments (SSDs) and housing departments

- Voluntary or charitable organizations

- Commercial or 'private' organizations

- Health services

provide community services in a way which is more flexible and responsive to the needs of individuals and their carers.

Local authority service provision – statutory or discretionary?

Statutory services are those which an Act of Parliament has put a duty upon the authority to provide under certain circumstances. The authority is permitted to provide discretionary services but is under no obligation to do so. Table 13.1 summarizes those statutory and discretionary services provided by local authorities for the elderly and the disabled. It can be seen that the elderly have a right to many services only by virtue of their disability. In this context 'disability' refers to 'persons who are blind, deaf or dumb or are

Table 13.1: Statutory (S) and discretionary (D) services provided or commissioned by local authorities for elderly and disabled people

	Elderly	Disabled
Information about services	D	S
Identification of those in need of services	D	S
Assessment of social, education and housing needs	–	S
Assessment of carers' ability to continue	–	S
Visiting and advisory services and social work support	D	D
Practical assistance at home	S	S
Aids and equipment	–	S
Meals at home or elsewhere	D	S
Recreational/educational facilities in/outside home	D	S
Transport to services provided by the authority or similar services	D	S
Occupational activities	–	D
Social rehabilitation	–	D
Telephone: assistance with provision	–	S
Facilities for taking holidays	–	S
Free or subsidized travel, if qualify for concessions	–	S
Home adaptations	D	S
Residential accommodation which is 'not otherwise available to them'	S	S
Nursing home care (with health authority approval)	D	D

substantially or permanently handicapped by illness, injury or congenital deformity, or who are suffering from a mental disorder as defined by the Mental Health Act'. More recently the interpretation has been extended to include 'people who are partially sighted or hard of hearing'. There is no requirement for such people to be registered as disabled.

Home-help service

The provision of home helps to new mothers was empowered by the Maternity and Childcare Act 1918. It was extended to the frail elderly in 1944 becoming mandatory in 1968 and as such has been one of the cornerstones of community care of the elderly. Over recent years, the role of home-help services has evolved to reflect the changing needs of an increasingly old and frail population. The traditional domestic duties of home helps involved general house-work and shopping and were most often provided on a once- or twice-weekly basis, virtually on demand. Increasing need for regular personal care such as washing, dressing and toiletting has necessitated new types of carers: care attendants, bath attendants and generic home care workers. With increasing demand for packages of care comprising several visits per day, seven days a week, the consequent pressure on resources in many areas has all but eradicated the traditional home help, and placed a greater reliance on commercial home-shopping services. The greater use of private sector providers of home-care services prompted by the Community Care Act, together with a tendency for authorities to charge commercial rates for these services, has increasingly blurred the boundaries between the private and public sectors.

Meals provision

'Meals on wheels' – the delivery of a hot meal direct to the home – were developed in the 1940s in response to the problems created by the Blitz in London and, from their inception, were run by the voluntary sector. In 1962, local authorities were empowered to develop their own meal services and today many still rely on voluntary organizations, such as Women's Royal Voluntary Service (WRVS) and Age Concern, for their local provision. Over recent years, the types of meal and mode of presentation have diversified catering for ethnic (e.g. Kosher, Asian, Afro-Caribbean) and medical (e.g. diabetic, gluten-free, pureed) requirements. Some authorities minimize distribution costs by providing bulk frozen meals to be heated by steamer or microwave. Luncheon clubs provide an alternative for those who are able to leave their homes, and they also have an important social function.

Aids and adaptations

'Aids' (to daily living) are the equipment used by people with disability to overcome their difficulty managing certain day-to-day tasks. Where such equipment forms part of the fixtures and fittings of the home they are referred to as (home) 'adaptations'.

Aids relating to mobility are the most ubiquitous. They include walking sticks, frames, trolleys and wheelchairs as well as non-slip mats and raised chairs, beds and toilet seats. 'Monkey poles', rope ladders and mattress variators can help aid bed mobility. The reduced reach of the older person can be overcome by use of a 'helping hand' and aids to putting on stockings. Disability from arthritic hands may be minimized by use of special taps, cooker knobs, jar-opening devices and thick-handled cutlery. Amplifiers for telephones and television can help those with hearing difficulties. Non-slip mats and bath seats aid bathing. Adaptations to the home may include fitting of grab rails and stair rails or ramps to aid wheelchair access. Accessible bathing and toilet facilities may be installed as may stair lifts. The frail elderly are less likely to obtain major adaptations. They more commonly make do with rearrangements to their living space which may eliminate the need to use stairs and minimize the need to walk by creating a 'bed-sit' within the home with commode toilet facilities.

Depending on individual circumstances an assessment for aids will be made either by the local authority SSD or health authority staff and in many places a common pool of equipment is maintained. The disabled living foundation provides useful advice on hire and purchase of most equipment.

Box 13.3: Features to consider in emergency alarms

- Trigger type: pendant, clipped to clothing, wrist strap

- Who alerted?: emergency centre, named helper(s) direct

- How alerted?: with or without direct speech link

- Options: sensors to warn of fire, hypothermia or burglary

Alarm systems

A wide selection of emergency alarm systems is available to older people who wish to have the security of knowing they can contact someone in an emergency, ranging from the fixed cord-pull systems traditionally provided in sheltered accommodation, to body-worn devices. Alarm systems may be provided by the local council or else can be privately purchased or rented (see Box 13.3).

Carer support

A variety of services is available to carers to help ease the burden of care. There is considerable diversity of provision but the major types include the following:

- Sitting services run by SSDs and voluntary organizations. These provide occasional or regular breaks for carers.

- Care attendant schemes such as those provided by Crossroads schemes. These aim to afford relief to carers by providing a flexible, tailored service.

- Counselling for carers. There are a number of examples of schemes jointly financed by SSDs and local voluntary bodies.

- Day care (see below), as well as fulfilling a major social function, is an excellent method of providing regular respite to a carer.

- Respite care. A complete break for the carer may be provided on an intermittent or regular basis. This usually entails temporary care in a residential or nursing home setting, or community hospital. Otherwise sufficient help may be provided in the client's home.

Transport

To the older person, loss of mobility outside the home is often a major cause of social isolation. The services available range from those which facilitate continued driving to the provision of transport for the severely disabled.

Driving

Refresher driving courses are available from major schools of motoring and 'Car confidence holidays' from SAGA Holidays. Mobility Advice and Vehicle Information Service (MAVIS) provides advice on simple low-cost adaptations to cars for people with disability. Advice to older drivers is available from the Department of Transport. Parking permits for those with disability are available through the orange-badge scheme.

Public transport

A variety of concessions are available for elderly and disabled people.

Door-to-door transport

Social cars are provided in some areas by local branches of voluntary organizations such as Women's Royal Voluntary Service (WRVS) and British Red Cross Society. Information on local schemes may be obtained via the National Council for Voluntary Organisations.

Dial-a-ride schemes provide local transport for those who are unable to use public transport due to disability. There is usually a need to book in advance.

Community transport is locally provided flexible transport, often run by voluntary groups.

Taxi card schemes are available to permanently disabled people throughout most of Greater London and offer large concessions on regular fares.

Social and recreation facilities

Day care in the form of luncheon clubs, social clubs and day centres may be organized by local authorities, voluntary organizations or religious and other cultural groups. Day centres usually take people for a whole day and provide transport. They may be attached to residential care homes forming community 'resource centres' and increasing use is being made of private sector provision. In many areas it has been recognized that the greatest need lies with the frailest individuals and the service has been designed to cater for this group's needs including suitable transport, the provision of health care input such as physiotherapy and chiropody, and the availability of specialist day care for those with dementia.

For those who are housebound, there are mobile reading library services, talking newspapers and social visiting schemes. A large number of specialist holidays are available to the elderly and disabled, information about which may be obtained from the Holiday Care Service.

Housing services

Repairs and adaptations

The elderly occupy a disproportionately large share of this country's unsuitable and substandard housing. They may also have changing housing needs due to the development of disability.

A wide variety of grants and loans are available, both mandatory and discretionary to cover minor works, housing renovation and provision of disabled facilities. It is a complex area, but advice and assistance is available from a number of sources including Care and Repair Ltd, which provides locally based home improvement housing agency services, sometimes known as 'Staying Put'.

Sheltered housing

This typically refers to privately purchased or rented accommodation arranged in a group of self-contained flats with a resident warden, an alarm system and some communal facilities, such as a residents' lounge, guestroom and laundry. Sheltered housing is commonly perceived to be a natural progression from totally independent living for elderly people with increasing frailty. However many schemes do not provide a greater level of personal support than can be provided in existing accommodation and the major consideration should be the quality of accommodation and social needs. Increasingly, schemes are available which provide extra help (extra care sheltered housing). The Elderly Accommodation Council maintains a national database of all forms of private, voluntary and charity accommodation for older people.

Keeping warm

The vulnerability of the elderly to hypothermia during cold weather is well recognized and a wide array of services are available to minimize the risk. Various (mostly) discretionary government loans and grants known collectively as the Social Fund are available for those eligible for Income Support and unable to pay themselves. They include budgeting loans, crisis loans, community care grants and cold weather payments. The Home Energy Efficiency Scheme (HEES) is available to all householders aged over 60 years and provides grants for loft, pipe, and water tank insulation and draught proofing. Council grants may be available for repairs and renovations (see above) and the fuel utilities offer assistance in the form of pre-payment meters, monthly budget schemes and flexible payments.

Financial advice and assistance

A number of Social Security benefits are available to older people or their carers (see Box 13.4). Additional benefits such as Disability Living Allowance and Independent Living Fund are available to those who develop their disability before the age of 66 years. Advice on benefits is available from the local Benefits Agency (social security) offices, and local offices of the Citizen's Advice Bureau and Age Concern.

Box 13.4: Main Social Security benefits available to older people and their carers

---

- **Income support:** A means-tested weekly paid benefit for those with a low income and limited savings

- **Attendance allowance:** A benefit for people disabled after the age of 65 years who, because of disability or illness, need (but are not necessarily receiving) help with personal care or supervision from another person. It is paid at a higher rate for those who need care by day and night

- **Invalid care allowance:** Available to people who claim before age 65 years and who spend 35 hours or more per week looking after someone who receives Attendance Allowance or certain other benefits

---

The legal arrangements available for managing financial affairs are summarized in Box 13.5. A concise summary is available from Age Concern (Fact sheet number 22: *Legal arrangements for managing financial affairs*).

Sensory impairment

Older people with significant visual or hearing impairment are eligible for the statutory services provided or commissioned by local SSDs.

The deaf/hard of hearing

Hearing tests and hearing aids are freely available within the NHS. Standard behind-ear or body-worn hearing aids are provided and maintained free of charge by hospital-based audiology departments. Local SSDs will usually convert doorbells to add flashing lights on ringing and may adapt telephones to make ringing and conversation more easily audible. The Advisory Committee on Telecommunications for Disabled and Elderly People (DIEL) produces an information pack on telephone services for use by older or disabled people and their helpers and it includes information on telephones for hard of hearing people.

Box 13.5: Legal arrangements for managing an elderly person's financial affairs

---

- **Agency:** An informal arrangement whereby disabled or ill people may appoint an 'agent' to collect their pension or social security benefits

- **Appointeeship:** In the case of temporary or permanent mental incapacity, a person may be appointed to claim and collect pension or social security benefits and to spend them on behalf of the claimant

- **Third party mandates:** A means by which disabled or ill people may nominate another individual to carry out bank or building society transactions on their behalf

- **Power of Attorney:** A legal document by which a person (donor) may appoint others (attorney) to act on their behalf. It is only valid while the donor is capable of giving instructions

- **Enduring Power of Attorney:** A power of attorney with which the attorney may continue to act on the donor's behalf after the donor becomes incapable of giving instructions

- **Court of Protection:** An Office of the Supreme Court, which protects the property and financial affairs of people who are incapable due to mental disorder. Following an application a receiver (usually a close relative) is appointed to manage the patient's affairs

---

The blind/partially sighted

People who are registered blind may be eligible for an additional disability premium if they receive Income Support, higher personal tax allowances and a modest television licence fee rebate. By virtue of their poor vision they may be eligible for the Attendance Allowance. In some areas there are concessionary rates for public transport. A wide range of special equipment and services is available to partially sighted people; including special telephones, talking book and newspaper services, kitchen aids, adapted games and writing frames. Often these services are managed by the local association for the blind and either accessed directly, or via the local SSD.

Urinary incontinence

Prevalence studies indicate that of people over 65 years living at home, 7–10% of men and 10–20% of women have urinary incontinence, yet traditionally the provision of continence services in the UK has been patchy and fragmented.

Advice

An initial source of assessment and advice is the community nursing service supported by specialist continence advisors (350 in the UK in 1995) who have a key role in education and in the planning and running of district continence services. Identifying treatable causes is paramount and preliminary medical assessment is the responsibility of the GP supported by specialist departments (e.g. urology and gynaecology) with access to investigative facilities, e.g. urodynamics assessment.

Product provision

Absorbent products, such as body-worn incontinence pads and bed pads, are not generally available on prescription. Health authorities have discretionary powers to provide them but there are major geographical variations in levels of provision. Some authorities employ regular delivery and soiled-product collection services. A wide range of collection devices, urinary catheters and drainage bags are available on prescription.

Laundry service

This may be provided by health and/or social services for heavily dependent incontinent people who experience regular wetting or soiling of bed linen or clothes. Alternatively, a washing machine and tumble drier may be provided and laundering carried out by home-care staff.

CHAPTER 14

Law and the older patient

Frank Fletcher, Carlyn Leslie and Peter Scott

The rapid growth in the proportion of the population over retirement age affects us all. This has led over the years to the introduction of laws related to the problems of older people and those with responsibilities towards them which has become an embryonic legal specialty in its own right.

This chapter introduces the most important and frequently encountered issues.

- Capacity.

- Consent to medical treatment.

- Advance statements regarding medical treatments ('Living Wills').

- Medical treatment at the end of life.

- Detention and treatment under the Mental Health Acts.

- Management of the patient's property.

Capacity

What is meant by capacity? It may be physical or mental and may be lost or impaired in old age, e.g. cataracts, stroke or intellectual impairment.

In a legal context, what matters is the patient's competence to do certain things that have legal consequences – consent to medical treatment, management of financial affairs, etc. – with the ability to understand the nature and effect of a decision and to make a reasoned judgement.

Increasingly, medical opinion on the capacity of elderly patients is sought by families, carers and solicitors. Before expressing an opinion, information should be obtained about the patient, his or her affairs and circumstances and about the nature, timing and effect of the proposed transaction.

Any view expressed should be restricted in its application to *that* transaction carried out at *that* time, as the older patient may be able to do some things but not others, or to do things at some times or in some circumstances but not others. A fresh judgement of capacity may be required *each time* an important decision needs to be taken. Lack of capacity to understand and consent to complex medical treatment does not infer lack of capacity to consent to more straightforward treatment; nor does lack of capacity to manage financial affairs infer lack of capacity to marry or to make a Will.

It is important to distinguish difficulty in communication (e.g. dysphasia, deafness or blindness) from diseases causing lack of capacity. The contemporary legal view of capacity was summarized recently by the Law Commission.

A person should be considered unable to take the decision in question (or decisions of the type in question) if he or she is unable to understand an explanation in broad terms and in simple language of the basic information relevant to taking it, or to retain the information long enough to take an effective decision.

A person should be considered unable to take the decision in question if he or she... can understand the information relevant to taking the decision but is unable because of mental disorder to make a true choice in relation to it, or ...is unable to communicate it to others who have made reasonable attempts to understand it.

Consent to medical treatment

A patient cannot be compelled to accept medical treatment. This can present problems with patients who have capacity to consent; the position is worse if capacity is doubtful or absent. Are doctors allowed to act on their own initiative and to what extent must they take account of the views of family or carers?

A patient's consent extends only to the treatment proposed and must be based on adequate information about its nature and likely effect and any other option open. While the doctor has a discretion as to the nature and extent of the information provided, he or she must draw all significant risks and benefits to the patient's attention in language the patient can understand.

Consent may be verbal or written, although surgery would normally only be conducted following written consent. Treatment must not normally extend beyond the limits of the patient's consent.

Consent to medical treatment is a personal decision for the patient: it *cannot* be delegated, whether to next-of-kin, a carer or social worker. While relatives and carers have no power to consent to or refuse treatment for a patient; they can help the doctor decide whether the proposed treatment is in the patient's best interests.

In assessing the patient's best interests, doctors should view the issue as they believe the patient would have done had the patient been competent to take the decision, rather than on the basis of their own subjective judgement. This approach can reflect the patient's known religious views and any anticipatory decision (e.g. 'Living Will') he or she may have made.

If doctors carry out treatment without consent, they may face criminal prosecution for assault and civil proceedings for damages. The law sometimes permits treatment where consent is lacking, or provides a defence for the doctor, as follows:

- the patient is unconscious, and emergency treatment may be given to save his or her life

- the patient lacks capacity to consent and the doctor considers the treatment to be in the patient's best interests

- the patient is detained under the Mental Health Acts and the treatment is authorized by the Acts

- the patient is suffering from a mental disorder such that he or she is a danger to himself or herself or others, when the defences of 'self defence' and 'reasonable force' are available to the doctor.

Patients who lack capacity may be disadvantaged because consent cannot be delegated. Recently, the High Court has developed a procedure enabling proposed treatment to be declared lawful. Although the court cannot give or refuse consent on a patient's behalf, it can declare that a particular treatment is lawful, if it is held to be in the patient's best interests. This procedure is intended for serious cases.

In Scotland, the system of 'tutors-dative' was recently revived. A tutor-dative is a person appointed by the court to take both personal and property decisions for a mentally incapacitated adult, including power to consent to medical treatment. Two medical certificates are required to support an application for a tutor.

Advance statements regarding medical treatment ('Living Wills')

A 'Living Will' is a document in which a patient specifically anticipates future medical treatment, and records his or her views about it.

In the US, several states have conferred legal effect on Living Wills by legislation. The position in the UK is less clear, where there is no such legislation, but the UK courts are increasingly taking a sympathetic view of them.

The versions in common use authorize treatments designed to ease pain and suffering, even if they result in earlier death, and the refusal of treatments designed to prevent or delay a 'natural' death. However, such a document cannot request a doctor to end a patient's life and any doctor who did so would be guilty of a criminal offence.

In April 1995, the BMA issued a Code of Practice 'Advance Statements about Medical Treatment' to provide guidance in dealing with them. Nevertheless, a number of problems remain:

• there is no agreed form

• lack of specificity may render it void

• have the particular circumstances contemplated by the statement, in fact, arisen?

• is the doctor responsible for the treatment aware of its existence?

• the possible interaction of the statement with life assurance policies, which may be related to the patient's death before, or survival to, a certain date

• difficulty in establishing that the statement has not been revoked

• uncertainty as to whether the statement is legally binding on the doctor.

The legal effectiveness of advance statements is not yet established. At present, all that can safely be said is that a Living Will is evidence of the patient's views and wishes when it was signed, and that the courts have favoured their implementation by prudent doctors who have consulted effectively with the patient's family and carers.

Medical treatment at the end of life

A doctor has no duty to preserve the patient's life at all costs. Enabling an incurably ill patient to die peacefully and with dignity is part of the doctor's role and may involve treatment that shortens life. If that treatment is designed to relieve the patient's suffering, the doctor will not be guilty of any offence, even if it results in the patient dying earlier than anticipated.

The law draws no distinction between withdrawing treatment already in progress and withholding treatment. There is, however, a clear distinction between allowing a patient to die and causing his death.

What if the patient refuses treatment? The doctor must ensure that the patient has:

• the capacity to make the decision

• not been unduly influenced by another person

• understood the nature and likely effect of the proposed treatment, and

• in his refusal, addressed the actual situation for which the treatment is proposed.

The position is particularly difficult where the patient lacks capacity. Because no other person can give consent, the proper course is to approach the courts for authority to adopt, withdraw or withhold a particular course of treatment. This procedure is only utilized in cases of persistent vegetative state, and is not usually applied to incurably ill older patients.

While family and carers may have strong views, they cannot take medical decisions on the patient's behalf. They may even have their own reasons for supporting or opposing a particular course, such as that life assurance policies will only pay out if the patient survives to, or dies before, a particular date; or that lifetime gifts made by the patient may be taxable unless he or she survives them by a specified period.

Compulsory detention and treatment

The patient's normal autonomy in regard to medical treatment is sometimes overruled by law, either in the public or the patient's interest.

Mental Health Act 1983

This Act applies to all patients suffering from 'mental disorder'. We will confine ourselves to the following aspects of the Act's application:

• compulsory admission and detention

• consent to treatment

- appeals

- guardianship.

Compulsory admission and detention

Section 2 provides that a patient may be compulsorily admitted to and detained in hospital *for assessment*, if his mental disorder is of a nature or degree warranting that detention and that it is in the interest of his health and safety or necessary for the protection of others. Compulsory detention is referred to as 'sectioning' the patient. Detention for assessment must be recommended by two doctors, can endure for up to 28 days and may not be renewed. Certain forms of treatment may be given during the detention, subject to the consent to treatment provisions.

Section 3 provides for the compulsory admission and detention of patients *for treatment*. Again the recommendation of two doctors is required, and these must contain particulars and reasons explaining why the necessary conditions have been met or are applicable. This authority lasts for six months but can be renewed a further six months in the first instance, but only if the requirements continue to be met. These requirements are more stringent than for a Section 2 admission.

Section 4 contains provisions for *emergency* admission for assessment. An application can be made by an approved social worker, or by the patient's nearest relative. It requires to be supported by only one doctor who has previous acquaintance with the patient. Emergency admissions are valid for 72 hours from admission, but then expire unless a second medical recommendation has been received.

A 'section' authorizes the patient's removal to hospital within 14 days, or in emergency cases 24 hours, from the time of the patient's last medical examination. It confers power to enter premises, and the patient is effectively in custody while being taken to hospital.

Consent to treatment

The consent to treatment provisions of Part IV of the Act apply to most *detained* patients, and specify the requirements for various treatments. Sections 57 and 58 regulate the administration of therapy, including ECT.

Appeals

Appeals by patients and their relatives against decisions under the Acts are dealt with by Mental Health Review Tribunals (MHRT). Where authority for detention has been renewed, the case must be referred every three years. The Secretary of State may also refer cases to a MHRT at any time.

Guardianship

Guardianship is a less severe form of compulsion, and is therefore more likely to be helpful in the case of older patients in the community. It applies to those with mental disorder who need supervision (e.g. those who fail or refuse to take their medication or neglect themselves) but who do not require compulsory admission.

Two doctor's certificates are required in support of an application for guardianship. The guardian may be the local social services authority or any individual.

The guardian's powers are limited to:

- requiring the patient to live at a specified place

- requiring the patient to attend at specified times and places for medical treatment, training or work

- requiring access to be given, at the patient's residence, to any medical practitioner, social worker or other person specified by the guardian.

The guardian cannot make personal decisions for the patient, such as consenting to medical treatment nor can compulsory treatment be given. Guardianship lasts for six months, but can be renewed for a further six months and annually thereafter.

The National Assistance Act 1948 S. 47

This provision can secure the necessary care and attention for persons who:

> are suffering from grave chronic disease or, being aged, infirm or physically incapacitated, are living in insanitary conditions and unable to devote themselves, or are not receiving from others, proper care and attention.

The 'designated medical officer' is empowered to remove that person to a place of safety if he or she considers this to be in the patient's best interests (or to prevent injury or serious nuisance to others).

A social worker must apply to the appropriate court for an order to remove the patient to a suitable hospital or local authority home for up to three months.

For urgent cases, emergency orders can be made but are only effective for three weeks.

Management of the patient's property

Some elderly patients become unable to manage their own affairs and doctors need to be aware of the options available for management of the patient's property by family, carers or professional advisors.

Informal methods

The extent of third-party management required depends on the extent of the incapacity and the sums involved. In cases of physical infirmity or mild dementia, informal methods may be sufficient. For example, calling on the goodwill of the patient's bank manager to permit a son or daughter to operate the patient's account. For patients of modest means, these may be the only cost-effective options available.

However, most informal methods of management (and even some of the statutory ones), whilst inexpensive and fairly easily arranged, involve little or no supervision, with the resultant risk of abuse or embezzlement.

Formal methods

Trusts

In wealthier families trusts may be created to provide for family members. Because the trust property is in the hands of trustees, the patient's incapacity does not affect its administration.

Powers of Attorney

More commonly, a patient's affairs are administered under a power of attorney. An agent ('attorney') is appointed by the patient to manage his affairs. So long as the patient had capacity to grant the power in the first place, the attorney's authority can now endure until the patient's death, notwithstanding the patient's subsequent loss of capacity. More than one attorney may be appointed, either to act together or separately.

In England and Wales, legislation requires the use of a statutory style of wording and the Power must be registered with the Court of Protection if the granter subsequently loses capacity. Thereafter, the attorney's powers are more limited and they are subject to the supervision of the Court.

In Scotland, there is no statutory style, no requirement for registration and no supervision of the attorney's actions, either before or after the patient's incapacity.

Such powers are a quick, cheap and private means of administration and allow the patient to choose who will look after their affairs on their incapacity. Because the patient must have capacity to grant the deed, doctors may frequently be asked to certify the patient's capacity for that purpose.

Attorneys must not allow their interests to conflict with those of the patient.

Receivership (curatory)

Where a patient lacks capacity to grant a power of attorney, the only alternative may be the appointment of a Receiver (in Scotland, a Curator).

In England and Wales, anyone with a relevant interest (e.g. a child, friend, carer, solicitor or social worker) may apply to the Court of Protection, under the provisions of Part VII of the Mental Health Act 1983, for the appointment of a 'Receiver'.

The Court must be satisfied that the patient is incapable, 'by reason of mental disorder', of managing his or her own affairs, before it will make an appointment. The patient's usual medical advisor will be asked for a report. Notice of the proceedings is served on the patient's closest relatives and also on the patient himself, unless this would cause him distress. A report on the suitability of the proposed Receiver is required, and the Receiver must usually take out a fidelity bond, to safeguard the patient's estate from maladministration or embezzlement.

The Receiver's authority is restricted to the patient's property, including costs of the patient's food, clothing, recreation and medical costs. The

Receiver is expected to consult the patient's doctor, social worker and carers as necessary, but has no real power over personal decisions including consent to medical treatment.

Patients are not allowed to manage their own affairs, though arrangements can be made for some handling of small sums, such as state benefits, or operation of a small bank account. The Receiver requires the Court's authority for certain acts, such as spending or investing capital or making gifts from the patient's property.

In Scotland, similar arrangements exist through the 'Curatory' system. The person appointed is a 'curator bonis'. The appointment is usually made in the Sheriff Court and thereafter the curator is subject to the supervision of the 'Accountant of Court'.

Further reading

Ashton G (1995) *Elderly People and the Law.* Butterworths, London.

Brazier M (1992) *Medicine, Patients and the Law* (2nd edn). Penguin, London.

Griffiths A and Roberts G (eds) (1995) *The Law and Elderly People* (2nd edn). Routledge, London.

Greengross S (ed.) (1989) *The Law and Vulnerable Elderly People.* Age Concern, London.

BMJ Publishing Group (1995) *Advance Statements about Medical Treatment.* BMJ Publishing Group, London.

McDonald A (1992) *Law and the Elderly.* Monograph 110 of the Social Work Monographs series. Social Work Monographs, Norwich.

Ward AD (1990) *The Power to Act.* Scottish Society for the Mentally Handicapped, Scotland.

CHAPTER 15

Medical ethics in community care

Donald Portsmouth

Older people have equal rights together with their younger fellow citizens for health care appropriate to their needs. That they do not always enjoy those rights underlines the need to examine the moral issues inherent in their care.

Medical practice is a moral exercise and doctors and their colleagues in the health care team are moral agents. Ethics is the study of moral choices and medical ethics is concerned with moral choices in medicine.

Ethical decisions are so closely associated with clinical decisions that they are usually not seen as separate from them. Doctors, however, can readily recognize what they consider to be unethical but they may not be so ready to define what is ethical, or indeed why it is considered so.

There has been a great upsurge in interest in medical ethics in the last three decades but despite this, it is still only just creeping into the syllabus in undergraduate medical education. Many doctors then will feel adrift on a chartless sea when ethical issues are discussed and such a situation tends to give rise to idiosyncratic and *ad hoc* decision making.

When a medical decision is challenged, doctors tend to retreat behind their professional armour and act defensively. Such a situation impairs the doctor–patient relationship which is the foundation of good practice. It is not usually on grounds of technical medical knowledge or opinion but on its appropriateness for a particular patient's circumstances and desires that a challenge is made. Such a challenge may represent a conflict between the patient's values and those of the doctor. Medical practitioners are so accustomed to making value judgements as part of their clinical practice that they may not be aware of the validity of the values they are using. It is usually assumed that they are understood as the agreed values of medical practice itself and do not need analysis.

Medical ethics has a long history dating from the time of Hippocrates (460–370 BC). The oath he described has been an icon for medicine ever since, though largely ignored in recent times. Jonsen has described the history of medical ethics to the present day starting with the Hippocratic code which emphasized competence in medical practice.[1] He follows its course through the spirit of compassion exemplified by the Good Samaritan to the 'noblesse oblige' spirit of condescension of Thomas Percival, the nineteenth-century Manchester physician and author of the first modern textbook of medical ethics. This condescension is in the manner of the eighteenth-century 'Enlightenment' and the duty inherent in serving the sick.

More recently, Osler described the humanities as the 'Hormones of Medicine'. Jonsen takes this analogy further by describing ethics as the 'Hormones of Medicine', in that they facilitate medical endeavour.

Medical ethics has been influenced by utilitarianism and deontological approaches, described by Beauchamp and Childress.[2] They define four principles as a framework for ethical decision-making which are now widely accepted as providing guidance to health care workers when formulating the solution to an ethical problem.

1 Beneficence.

2 Non-maleficence.

3 Respect for autonomy.

4 Justice.

Beauchamp and Childress' four principles

The first two principles will be familiar as they are rooted in the ethical tradition of medicine. Autonomy, however, is less familiar and has advanced in stature in recent times. Respect for autonomy counter-balances the traditional paternalism in the doctor–patient relationship and is promoted by political initiatives affecting social life in general and health care in particular.[3] It is easy to ignore or marginalize in elderly care, as the vulnerability of old people often renders them hostages to fortune.

Justice speaks of fairness in the allocation of resources. The elderly are sometimes targeted as a group for whom some advances in medical techniques are inappropriate. Where the old ethics spoke of individuals, the new ethics more often sees individuals as members of a group with common characteristics. The elderly, however, are by no means a uniform group and share as much diversity as do those of other ages, if not more.

Solving ethical dilemmas is not easy. Recourse to the four principles, however, can identify the factors involved in any particular situation. The weight given to each principle requires reflection and discussion and must be based on the realities of the elderly patient's situation.

The commonest error in clinical geriatrics is to seek a solution before defining a problem. This is as true of ethical dilemmas as it is of clinical. Determining the truth is often the most difficult part of the exercise. Elderly patients in the community in need of medical attention are often surrounded by a coterie of interested parties, some are relatives, some are not; some are supportive, some are not. Any may provide subjective views of the situation. Even professionals may not be truly objective and can allow their hearts to rule their heads.

This calls for patience, clear-thinking and above all a desire to seek out facts on which to base decisions. Facts about the history, facts about functional ability; facts about the patient's

personal situation and desires. It is so easy to be misled and a degree of suspicious inquisition is fully justified in establishing the basis for decision-making. Indeed, without a knowledge of the facts, practitioners cannot discharge their responsibility for which in any event they will be held accountable.

None of the four principles should be used habitually to trump the others. Autonomy perhaps is the one most likely to be used in this way – it must always be remembered that one person's autonomy may obstruct the exercise of another's. This is particularly so in elderly care in the community where to exercise autonomy may depend on the support and sacrifice of others. Gillon describes the use of the four principles with attention to their scope of application, a very valuable contribution.[4]

The aims of elderly care

When discussing the management of an individual elderly patient it is vital that members of the health care team share common aims. If the team is practised at working together, the aims may not be debated but nonetheless conflict can arise in particular circumstances. So complex are the situations of some elderly people in the community that the problems they give rise to appear insoluble. Time and patience are necessary to unravel the tangled web step-by-step before the path to a satisfactory solution is found. This is where undue emphasis given to one of the four principles can distort the situation and lead to expedient solutions, perhaps resolving an immediate crisis but leaving a 'time-bomb' of problems for the future.

Risk-taking

Risk-taking is inherent in the practice of geriatric medicine. Indeed, without taking calculated risks it is likely that the quality of an elderly person's life is unnecessarily restricted. To calculate the risk involved in either a particular style of living, or a particular undertaking as well as a proposed medical or surgical procedure, requires the striking of a balance between beneficence and non-maleficence. Possible benefits and possible harms are always to be borne in mind but in the end it is the autonomous choice of the patient that must be paramount in circumstances where there is no doubt about the choice and that it is based on adequate information and understanding.

Nonetheless, if the choice seriously affects the interests and autonomy of others there must be room for discussion and compromise. Just as the elderly person's autonomy commands respect, so does that of the 'significant others'. Professional staff ought never to perform an act they believe to be wrong or inappropriate because they are requested to do so by their patient or client.

Vulnerability

Many elderly people are vulnerable because of physical or mental frailty or because their social circumstances are inappropriate for them. Such is fertile ground for paternalism which is not recognized as such as it is disguised and justified as beneficence. It is not so much frailty itself that gives rise to vulnerability but the loss of independence it may bring. Resulting dependence for essential support renders the elderly subject to the interest of others. Such interests may conflict with the interests of the old person. It is when older people are seen as part of a group rather than as individuals who are old that their interests are most likely to be marginalized. Ethical practice must always be centred on the particular person as they are and not as they appear to be in reflection of the commonly held stereotypes of ageing.

Capacity

Critical to the exercise of autonomy is mental capacity, though casting doubt on the latter is a common reason for denying respect for the former. Personal autonomy grants the right to follow a self-chosen plan based on choice. Clearly there are limits to this exercise and pragmatism demands recognition of those limits in individual cases. These should not be imposed, however, with the object of placing undue limitations on the exercise of choice. Freedom from such influence is inherent in the concept of autonomy.

It can of course be an autonomous choice to surrender autonomy in a particular situation to others but this should never be assumed. More

often casting doubt on an older person's capacity for thought and action corrupts the process of providing care. Assessment of mental capacity is an important part of the clinical approach to old people. When the question is the capacity for decision-making it must be seen as task specific. A person may be incompetent to make choices in some areas of his or her life because of not having the capacity to understand the facts, weigh their significance and make appropriate choices and decisions. However, in other aspects of life, if properly informed, such a person may well maintain the capacity for autonomous decision-making. This has been upheld in the case of Re C; the case of a 68-year-old schizophrenic man who despite severe delusions was considered capable of refusing a proposed amputation of his leg for gangrene.[5]

The Law Commission report on Mental Incapacity recommends that there should be a presumption against lack of capacity and that any question whether a person lacks capacity should be decided on the balance of probabilities (para 3.2).[6] This is sound clinical precedent too and as it is the doctor who is usually asked to provide an opinion on capacity, it should be the guideline of good practice.

However, it is often borderline cases where judgement is difficult. Perhaps it is where capacity appears to be adequate but where it is not linked to a sense of reality that the hardest situations arise. Patience, repeated examination and the exercise of sensitivity are more than ever necessary in this situation and sometimes a patient's decision simply has to be put to the test with all precautions taken to prevent harm from possible risks.

Interfaces with other agencies

Traditional medical ethics was based on the doctor–patient relationship on the basis that this was a 'one-to-one' encounter. The reality of contemporary practice with elderly patients is that this is seldom so.

The interests of third parties can distort the interface between doctor and patient and the ability to control the debate is an essential attribute. To do this requires a knowledge of ethical principles and experience in their practical expression.

Strategies to avoid ethical conflict are part of a clinician's armamentarium and demand considerable sensitivity and skill. The recent NHS reforms and community care initiatives have changed the ground rules and shifted the balance of power. Though overtly the patient's interests are accorded priority, in effect they are subject to quasi-commercial pressures arising from the 'purchaser-provider' division. Constant vigilance and appropriate criticism and comment are essential as the doctor may be the only person with an overall and disinterested view. 'Holding the ring' in the debate which inevitably gives rise to conflict in long acknowledged values, is a challenge that has to be met.

The patient in his or her own house has the advantage of being on home territory. This tilts the balance of power to the patient's advantage and many elderly people instinctively appreciate this. To insist, however, on treatment at home rather than at hospital when the latter is deemed indicated can result in inappropriate use of resources, challenging the principles of justice and fairness to others and also exposing the doctor to unjustifiable risk-taking.

Conversely, those who demand treatment in hospital when home management appears the better option may also be guilty of misusing resources which by definition are always finite.

Pressure from the informal carers by threatening to withdraw their involvement and thus precipitate admission to hospital or residential home has to be recognized and faced. The question 'who is the patient?' has to be asked and the answer analysed.

Of course, the carers may be at the limit of their resources or even beyond and this must be recognized. They may have been subjected to undue pressure and the reality of the situation must be presented to the individual being cared for. In these circumstances, it is essential for the health care team to share a common view, achieved by discussion, or else the situation will get out of control and be subject to the chance of circumstances and expedient decision-making.

Of course, community care may fail or indeed be inappropriate for a patient decreed suitable for discharge from hospital. Good communication between professional staff, patient and carers, the basis of all ethical decision-making, is essential in these circumstances.

'End-of-life' decisions

Most people would agree that if possible, home is the best place to die. For many, however, it is not practicable and this can lead to lack of recognition of the elderly person's values and desires. To overcome this problem is the motive behind the move to promote advance directives.

The British Medical Association has recently published a code of practice for advance statements about medical treatment.[7] This sets out the principles of such statements which already have statutory recognition in the US. The Law Commission has recommended similar status in the UK but a government decision on the issue is currently awaited, though there is arguably case law in their favour.

Advance statements promote the principle of informed consent to treatment by making an anticipatory declaration in general terms, or even by specifying treatments that would be unacceptable. While everyone would agree that informed consent to treatment is a principle that must be upheld for the elderly as much as for other age groups, there are problems inherent in withdrawing such consent in advance. The aim is clearly to be provided with appropriate comfort, care and pain relief but to avoid being subjected to life-sustaining techniques that may result in the prolongation of dying rather than the continuance of worthwhile life. Of course, if patients make their wishes known to their family doctor in advance and these are noted in the clinical record for passing on to appropriate colleagues at the appropriate time, such declarations may be unnecessary. Perhaps this is a counsel of perfection and an indication in general terms without excluding specific treatments would seem to be unexceptional.

There is as yet no firm data from North America about the effect of advance statements on clinical practice and it would seem prudent to await such evidence before giving them statutory force which may in effect compromise a patient's best interests.

There is as yet no accepted legal framework except for individual judicial consideration, for health care decisions concerning an incompetent adult to be made by another person. The guidelines remain as the 'best interests' of the patient coupled with the doctor's 'duty of care'. Where difficult decisions have to be made it is good practice to consult colleagues for their opinion but this is not commonly done in the UK.

Difficult decisions have to be made in cases of terminal illness in the elderly with regard to sedation, pain relief and the provision of food and fluids. Legal judgements on these matters can easily be misconstrued. The decision in the case of Tony Bland[8] was specific to the so-called permanent vegetative state which in many important respects is different from the situation of the elderly patient with advanced cerebrovascular disease or Alzheimer's dementia. Refusing treatment, including food and water is legitimate if a patient is competent to do so. Withholding or withdrawing treatment is legitimate if they are not considered to be in the patient's best interests.

A difficult decision is in the case of the incompetent patient with a secure means of providing nutrition, such as perendoscopic gastrostomy tube. In the past, with nasogastric tubes which in practice were less reliable, decisions were often made by default. Now they have to be made definitively and are more difficult as a result. Consultation, discussion and respect for the patient's interests would lead to appropriate management.

Resource allocation

Resources are often considered as materials such as drugs, dressings, equipment and buildings. The doctor and his team are the most valued resource, however, in health care terms and the allocation of sufficient time and attention to elderly patients is inherent in good geriatric practice. Too often doctors belittle their own input when they consider a problem to be more social than medical. In truth there is no social problem concerning the elderly without a medical component just as there is no medical problem that does not call for ethical consideration as well.

References

1 Jonsen AR (1990) *The new medicine and the old ethics.* Harvard University Press, London.

2 Beauchamp TL and Childress JF (1994) *Principles of biomedical ethics* (4th edn). Oxford University Press, Oxford.

3 Department of Health (1991) *The Patient's Charter.* Department of Health, HMSO, London.

4 Gillon R (1994) Medical ethics: Four principles plus attention to scope. *BMJ* **309**:184–8.

5 (1994) Re C: adult; refusal of medical treatment. *AELR* **1**:89.

6 (1995) *Mental Incapacity.* Law Commission Report No. 231. HMSO, London.

7 BMJ Publishing Group (1995) *Advance Statement About Medical Treatment.* BMJ Publishing Group, London.

8 Kennedy I and Grubb A (1994) *Medical Law, Text with Materials.* Butterworths, London, pp. 1217–38.

Key points

- Medical ethics is concerned with moral choices in medical practice
- Determining the truth is the basis for ethical as well as clinical decisions
- The four principles can be used as guidelines for shaping an ethical debate
- The health care team should share common values and aims for elderly patients
- Recognizing the vulnerable elderly patient is a prerequisite to ethical decision-making
- An elderly patient should be presumed to have capacity unless it is proved otherwise
- Good communications with patients and their relatives is essential for an understanding of their values

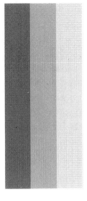

CHAPTER 16

Older people in ethnic minority groups

Alistair Ritch

In recent years there has been a growing awareness of issues involving ageing, race and ethnicity. As many immigrants of the 1950s reach retirement age, it has become apparent that the disadvantages of growing old are enhanced by racial discrimination, social deprivation, shortened life expectancy, greater morbidity and unequal access to health and social services.

It is important to distinguish between race and ethnicity, although there are no simple definitions of either. Race suggests differences based on physical appearance. An ethnic group is characterized by a sense of identity and implies a common geographical origin, language, religion or distinctive traditions. The two ethnic minority groups which have been the subject of the most study in this country will be referred to as Asian and Afro-Caribbean. The latter includes those people from the West Indies of African origin. All who originate from the Indian subcontinent are collectively described as Asian, although it must be recognized that there are ethnic differences between people from India, Pakistan and Bangladesh. Box 16.1 lists the breakdown of the major ethnic groups in the UK.

Demography

In the 1991 Census, 5.5% of the total population described themselves as belonging to a group 'other-than-White'. Of these, 3% were 65 years and over while 15% were aged between 45 to 64 years. This compares with 17% and 22% respectively for the white population. A dramatic rise in the number of ethnic elders is forecast over the next 20 years. At present, they are on average younger than indigenous pensioners (see Table 16.1).

Box 16.1: Major ethnic groups in Great Britain as a percentage of all ethnic minority groups, from 1991 census

Indian	28%
Black Caribbean	17%
Pakistani	16%
Black African	7%
Bangladeshi	5%
Chinese	5%

Table 16.1: Age differences in older inner-city residents of West Birmingham

	White (%)	Asian (%)	Afro-Caribbean (%)
65–74 years	50	72	87
75–84 years	41	23	13
85+ years	9	5	0

Social concerns

Social deprivation

There is a greater concentration of ethnic minority population in the inner-city areas of London and the Metropolitan Counties. Ethnic elders in these situations experience the social deprivation associated with inner-cities, such as poverty, poor housing and high unemployment. These factors are likely to have more impact on their health profile than ethnicity.

Language

An inability to speak and understand English is a major barrier to communication among older Asians. Even the one out of ten Asians who can speak English are likely to have difficulty when communicating with health professionals. In such situations the services of a trained interpreter should be used. Furthermore, many older Asians are unable to read any language, including their mother tongue.

Household size

While the impression that Asians live in extended households holds true in general, it cannot be assumed in all circumstances. Although under 10% of older Asians live alone, this proportion appears to be rising and around a quarter of them have no family in Britain. Well over half of older Asians live in households with four or more other people, although this can lead to overcrowding, with a quarter sharing a bedroom with a person who is not their spouse (see Table 16.2). One exception to this pattern is those Asians who have come to Britain from East Africa who are more likely to live in a nuclear family.

Table 16.2: Household size of older inner-city residents in West Birmingham

	White (%)	Asian (%)	Afro-Caribbean (%)
1 person	43	7	24
2 persons	45	22	45
3–4 persons	8	12	26
5+ persons	4	59	4

As a result of the extended family situation, dependent older Asians have greater access to carers living within their own household giving rise to the belief that ethnic elders are always looked after by their families. Access to health care must not be denied because of this assumption that they can cope unaided. Some families may take on the caring role because the cultural attitudes prevailing in their local community expect it of them and they may feel unable to request the support they need.

Patterns of disease

Differences in patterns of disease between ethnic minority groups and the indigenous population are beginning to emerge. Immigrants are usually in better health compared with the population of the country they leave, although there will remain some influence of disease prevalent in their previous homeland. What is surprising is the high rate of so-called 'Western' disease. For instance, Asians and Afro-Caribbeans have a greater than expected prevalence of diabetes mellitus, while Asians suffer more coronary artery disease and Afro-Caribbeans more hypertension and stroke illness (see Box 16.2).

Box 16.2: Diseases more common in Asians and Afro-Caribbeans

Asians

- Diabetes mellitus
- Coronary artery disease
- Cataract
- Osteomalacia
- Tuberculosis
- Asthma

Afro-Caribbeans

- Hypertension
- Stroke
- Diabetes mellitus
- Tuberculosis

Information on older people is scanty but there appears to be an excess of older Asians discharged from hospital with a diagnosis of asthma, gastrointestinal bleeding, diabetes mellitus and myocardial infarction. More have had cataract surgery and more older Asians report impaired vision. Alcohol-related morbidity has been reported to be more common in Sikh men, although their religion forbids the use of alcohol. An increased prevalence of chronic disease was found in one study of Gujaratis in London, and a higher rate of arthritis detected among Asians in Birmingham. An awareness of the ethnic composition of the local population and hence of the health problems likely to be encountered will assist in the setting up of appropriate primary preventive strategies.

Very little is known about the mental health of older people in ethnic minority groups and no information is available on the impact of dementia. Assessment scales in current use are culturally inappropriate; most requiring a knowledge of British history. Furthermore, many older Asians are not conversant with their exact age and date of birth. Reports of less anxiety and depression among Asians have to be interpreted with caution since good communication is necessary for accurate diagnosis.

Hypertension and stroke

There is an increased prevalence of hypertension among Afro-Caribbeans and Africans in Britain and this includes older individuals. Hypertension is found in 25–35% of Afro-Caribbeans of all ages, compared with 15–20% of the indigenous population, and is responsible for an excess of deaths from stroke of the order of 76% for men and 110% for women, compared with the norm for England and Wales. Hypertensive Afro-Caribbeans are more likely to develop renal failure but have a lower incidence of coronary artery disease.

Hypertensive blacks in the US have been found to have an increased capacity to retain salt. This and the high salt-intake characteristic of Western societies may be the explanation for the increased prevalence of hypertension. It may also be responsible for suppressing renin release leading to significantly lower plasma levels found in hypertensive Afro-Caribbeans. Salt restriction plays an important role in management of older Afro-Caribbeans

and thiazides are the most effective first-line drugs. Following these, calcium-channel blockers will be more effective in reducing blood pressure than other classes of antihypertensives.

Coronary artery disease

There has been increasing interest in recent years with respect to coronary artery disease within the Asian population in Britain although the research to date is almost exclusively confined to those below pensionable age. For instance, the excess mortality resulting from coronary artery disease in adults up to the age of 70 years is 35% and 46% for Asian men and women respectively. This is the highest for any group within the population and is unique in showing no signs of improving. Asians have a myocardial infarction rate which is five times higher than the rest of the population and usually they have more extensive coronary artery atheroma.

The high prevalence cannot be explained by the usual risk factors for atheroma, such as smoking, hypertension or cholesterol levels. It is associated with a disturbance of glucose metabolism characterized by increased insulin resistance. Studies of plasma cholesterol levels have produced contradictory findings, though low density lipoproteins which show an inverse correlation with the presence of atherosclerosis may be lower in Asians. They appear to be highest in Afro-Caribbeans who have the lowest mortality from coronary artery disease of any ethnic group in Britain. Another possible explanation for the increased incidence in Asians is the widespread use in cooking of clarified butter (ghee), which contains potentially atherogenic cholesterol oxides.

Diabetes mellitus

Non-insulin dependent diabetes is present in around 5% of the indigenous population of Britain over the age of 40 years. It is at least twice as common in Asians and Afro-Caribbeans and has been recorded to be as high as 30% among Asians over 45 years in whom one-third had not previously been diagnosed as diabetic. There is an association with central obesity and insulin resistance in Asians. They are more likely to develop proteinuria and end-stage renal failure but less likely to have peripheral vascular disease or require amputation. Despite the connection between insulin resistance and coronary artery disease, they have not been shown to be more prone to angina or myocardial infarction than white diabetics.

Asian diabetics have been reported as having less well controlled plasma glucose levels. Social customs involving the consumption of certain types of food, such as sweetmeats, may contribute to this. There is a need for educational materials that are culturally appropriate, written in different languages and provided in alternatives to written text for those who are unable to read in any language.

Osteomalacia

Although the prevalence of rickets among Asian children in Britain has greatly diminished, osteomalacia remains more common in older Asian adults than in other sections of the population. It may account for the higher annual incidence of fractured neck of femur that has been found in Asian men in Leicestershire. Older Asians have been shown to have lower 25-hydroxyvitamin-D levels, to complain more of generalized pain and to have an altered gait. As they are at higher risk for developing osteomalacia, bone biochemistry should be checked in all those with symptoms suggestive of arthritis. The reasons for vitamin-D deficiency are multiple but include poor dietary intake, consumption of chapatis high in phytic acid and reduced exposure to sunlight. In addition, ageing results in a decline in photosynthesis of vitamin-D in the skin and in a reduction in renal function which impairs the production of the active metabolite of the vitamin.

Tuberculosis

The notification rate for tuberculosis in Asians is about 40 times greater than the indigenous population and mortality is increased by a factor of five. Afro-Caribbeans also have a three-fold increase in the incidence of this disease. Non-respiratory forms such as lymph node involvement are common in Asian adults. It is an example of disease relating to country of origin as it is more common in recent immigrants and those returning from holiday in their previous

homeland. However, there remains a strong link between tuberculosis and poverty in Britain. The socio-economic disadvantages of the inner-city, particularly overcrowded households, are responsible for maintaining a high prevalence of the disease among ethnic minority groups.

Functional ability

Attempts to compare disability between ethnic and indigenous elders have produced conflicting results varying from twice the level of disability among Asians, to no difference in an age controlled population. Cultural differences also play a confounding role when measuring activities of daily living. For instance, an older Asian man in an extended family would not be expected to be able to cook, while an older Asian woman would not go out alone, especially in an inner-city area. The response to chronic disease may vary and within some cultures families may become overprotective. Sufferers may expect help from within the family as a right and so not wish to co-operate with rehabilitation. A question was included in the 1991 Census about the presence of limiting long-term illness which restricted daily activities even if thought to be due to old age. Analysis by ethnic group for those of pensionable age revealed a slightly higher prevalence among the Asian groups (about 41%) and in Black Caribbeans (40%) compared to the White (36%) and Chinese (29%) groups. As the average age of the first two groups is likely to be lower than the White group, there is likely to be a higher level of disability at an earlier age among Asian and Afro-Caribbean pensioners.

Use and awareness of services

General practitioners

An increased consultation rate with the general practitioner (GP) within the preceding six months has been found for Asian patients, for example 92% compared with 63% of the older indigenous population. However, consultation rates within the inner-city are above 90% for all groups of the older population. There is no evidence that any increase in use is inappropriate and it is likely to

Table 16.3: Contact with health services for older residents in West Birmingham

	White (%)	Asian (%)	Afro-Caribbean (%)
GP	92	98	94
Dentist	52	34	62
Community nurse	14	3	11
Chiropodist	43	3	20
Physiotherapist	12	2	8

Table 16.4: Knowledge of community health services among older residents in West Birmingham

	White (%)	Asian (%)	Afro-Caribbean (%)
Health visitor	47	13	54
Community nurse	91	30	84
Auxiliary nurse	44	5	66
Psychiatric nurse	28	2	33
Chiropodist	94	10	87
Physiotherapist	80	14	67
Occupational therapist	33	1	23
Dietitian	78	13	84

be a reflection of poorer health. However, there may be a cultural element in terms of high expectations from medical contact and greater awareness of the GP service compared with other primary care services. Despite high use by Asians, satisfaction levels are no different from other patients. Indeed, white patients are more likely to leave the surgery with a prescription or follow-up appointment.

Community health services

By contrast, older Asians had very little contact with the community nursing services compared with Afro-Caribbeans and whites in the previous year (see Table 16.3). This was also true for those suffering from disability where it appeared to be due to lack of referral of Asian patients by their GPs. One explanation for this may be the stereotyped view that they will be cared for by their families. Another may be lack of awareness among Asians of all types of community nurses, including psychiatric nurses. When given an explanation of the role of the community nurse, they show a willingness to use the services if required. A similar lack of use and awareness occurs across the whole range of community services, including physiotherapy and chiropody. In comparison Afro-Caribbeans use services to the same extent as the white population and show the same degree of awareness (see Table 16.4).

Social services

There is an increasing body of evidence showing that little use is made by ethnic minority groups of community services provided by the local authority. This holds true across the whole range of provisions including home care, meals on wheels, luncheon clubs, day centres and respite care. The range of use for all ethnic groups is usually found to be less than 10% for home care and meals and frequently no Asian elders receive these services. Knowledge of their existence is likewise low, reflecting service use, with under one half not having heard of any of the community services. By contrast, the use of services by Afro-Caribbeans is low but knowledge of their existence is greater than Asians.

Although both groups have experienced problems when using services, only in Asians are these related to ethnicity, for instance communication difficulties and diet. When appropriate services are provided, often by voluntary groups, the take-up is usually high. However, older Asians see themselves as needing these less as they assume their families will provide the care they need. They are also less inclined to use home-care because of the lack of Asian home helps and have expressed concern over the type of food provided by meals on wheels.

Positive discrimination?

Because of the low use of health and social services, should specific services be set up to provide for the special needs of ethnic minority groups? Older Asians and Afro-Caribbeans do not themselves prefer separate provision although it would cater for many of their concerns such as diet and language. To date, the prevailing attitude has been that a common set of services should be provided for everyone to either use or reject. A more equitable approach would be to attempt to meet the individual needs of older people which would then include those in ethnic minority groups. This is particularly important for older groups who are immigrants and have had less opportunity and desire to assimilate into the host society.

Health authorities have been criticized for being slow to respond to health issues affecting ethnic minority groups. Both primary and secondary health care facilities remain inflexible resulting in unequal access and less favourable standards of care. The provision of specific services would be one way of achieving equity of access for everyone.

While emphasis has been placed on greater prevalence of disease and failure to meet health and social needs, individuals in ethnic minority groups should not be regarded as 'problems'. Rather greater awareness and understanding of differences should help towards developing a more sensitive approach to health care.

Key points

Ethnic minority groups:

- have a lower percentage of people aged over 75 years

- have a higher than average level of social deprivation

- have more extended families

- have higher rates of chronic disease, e.g. TB, diabetes, hypertension, coronary disease and stroke

- have higher levels of disability at an earlier age

- are poorly informed (often due to language problems) about, and underuse, health and social resources

Further reading

Atkin K and Rollings J (1993) *Community care in a multi-racial Britain.* HMSO, London.

Ebrahim S and Hillier S (1991) Ethnic minority needs. *Reviews in Clinical Gerontology* 1:195–9.

Hopkins A and Bahl V (1993) *Access to health care for people in black and ethnic minorities.* Royal College of Physicians, London.

Squires A (1991) *Multicultural health care and rehabilitation of older people.* Edward Arnold, London.

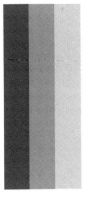

CHAPTER 17

Taking the Diploma in Geriatric Medicine

Bryan Moore-Smith

Founded in 1986, the Diploma of the Royal College of Physicians of London, copied in both Scotland and Ireland, encapsulates in its wide syllabus, demographic and social factors, the clinical aspects of old age and the administrative features of services in the UK.

The purpose of the diploma examination is to identify the holders as doctors who have special knowledge and expertise in the care of elderly people. It is currently primarily aimed at doctors in general practice in the UK but is open to aspiring specialists in any medical discipline serving older patients.

The diploma is of special significance for clinical assistants, hospital practitioners and staff-grade doctors working in non-consultant posts in departments of geriatric medicine.

Such recognized expertise among doctors contributes greatly to the standard of general practice in an ageing population in particular, as well as to the effectiveness and efficiency of departments of geriatric medicine. The closure of much long-stay NHS accommodation and its replacement by privately run alternatives requires assurances to the purchasers that the standards are acceptable. Medical officers to such establishments will more and more need to be able to demonstrate their knowledge and expertise to purchasers, frequently local authority departments of social services. The Association of Directors of Social Services is known to be increasingly concerned about this matter.

The standard required is high, and is assured both by the extent of the body of knowledge and, in the clinical examination, the emphasis on clinical skills and the ability to relate to elderly people. There is an average pass rate of 65% and holders of 'higher' qualifications, such as the MRCP, do not always automatically succeed at their first attempt.

Entry qualifications

The criteria are widely drawn and the examination is open to any qualified doctor, who either has held or is currently holding, a post approved for professional training in a department specializing in the care of the elderly, or who has had experience over a period of two years since qualification in which care of the elderly formed a significant part (Royal College of Physicians Regulations 1995).

The diploma may therefore be taken early in their careers by doctors who work in departments of elderly care, intending to enter general practice, and is particularly relevant for those in vocational training schemes for general practice whose rotations include such experience. Equally, established general practitioners (GPs) may well need to be able to demonstrate recognized expertise to purchasers. While not a requirement for those planning to be specialists in hospital in the care of elderly people, taking the diploma offers an opportunity to survey the body of knowledge in its entirety, and is perhaps of special importance for those intending to work in the psychiatry of old age.

Preparation for the examination

Read the syllabus. This is obtainable, as are past papers, from the Royal College of Physicians. Make sure you understand it. Note that the overall standard required is that of good quality primary care. Appreciate the emphasis placed on the synthesis of diagnostic and clinical examination skills with the planning of management strategies in the light of current arrangements in health and social services.

The syllabus contains three major divisions:

1 demographic and social factors

2 clinical aspects of old age

3 administrative features of services.

Of these, the largest part comes under heading 2. The subjects covered here include:

* age-associated changes in the major body systems

* preventative aspects in later life

* presentational problems in diagnosis

* specific clinical problems important in old age

* pharmacology and therapeutics in old people

* the principles of rehabilitation

* domiciliary care

* legal aspects

* clinical considerations

* terminal care.

All these themes may arise in the papers and during the course of the long- and short-case clinical examinations, as do demographic and social considerations and administrative features.

Current experience in the clinical examination and management of elderly patients is very important.

The examination

The examination consists of three parts which each carry equal marks. These are the written papers, the clinical long-case examination and the clinical short-cases examination.

The written papers are sat in March or April and in October and are held at the Royal College of Physicians. There are two written papers: Paper one lasts three hours in which 20 short note questions in five sections have to be answered. Each answer should be of about 100 words. All questions are to be attempted. The sections are devoted to broad topics such as the CNS, social factors, diseases of bone, drugs, gastrointestinal system, rehabilitation, cardiovascular system, etc.

Paper two contains two sections and lasts two-and-a-half hours, in which four questions are to be answered. In the first section there are two essay questions on broad topics, e.g. the effect of retirement on health. One of these is to be attempted. The second section contains one compulsory question, usually a narrative type question with four or five parts; sometimes it is on a single topic with specific sub-sections. After which there are three management problems of which two have to be answered.

The pattern of the second paper in particular is subject to a continuous process of amendment and evolution. Any major changes are notified to intending candidates.

The other two parts of the examination are clinical and are held at a variety of centres throughout England and Wales. They take place in May and December about six to eight weeks after the papers. Each clinical examination consists of a long case, and a series of short cases which may be interspersed with slides, videos and examples of physiotherapy and occupational therapy equipment. The long-case and the short-case material carry equal marks.

Written papers

In the papers, trends are evident in the short-note questions from those which fail less than 20% of candidates to those which fail more than 40%. In the less taxing group lie most questions on the gastrointestinal system, those on commonly used drugs, chest diseases and day-to-day biochemistry. More than 20% of candidates have difficulty with a range of questions on haematology, bone disease, the CNS, the cardiovascular system, the eye, skin conditions, hypnotics, L-dopa side-effects and social matters. Over 30% of candidates fail questions on ageing, a wide range of CNS subjects, the unstable bladder, rehabilitation and social aspects. More than 40% of candidates are unable to answer correctly questions on many features of rehabilitation, social aspects, many degenerative CNS conditions, and the non-catheter management of incontinence. It is apparent that candidates' knowledge is weakest in rehabilitation, social matters, the CNS (which accounts for many problems in the elderly population including such common things as stroke, depression and Parkinsonism), the ageing process and the promotion of continence.

The lists are not comprehensive. High fail rates lead to repeated questioning in subsequent examinations and concentration on weak areas while continuing to cover the whole syllabus over a period.

The other two main divisions of the syllabus tend to be covered, though not exclusively, in the demographic and wider social considerations by essays, and the administrative aspects through management problem questions.

Clinical examination

Although the papers are important, particularly to ensure that candidates cover the whole field of knowledge, the clinical examinations account for the highest proportion of failures. In preparing for the clinicals the *sine qua non* is active and recent experience in treating elderly patients. The candidate's approach to the patient, and to the carer if present, is crucial. Whenever possible, examiners take the candidate back to the long-case patient to observe the degree of rapport which has been achieved and the examination technique. Practice in examining and presenting patients before an audience is essential. The same considerations apply to the short cases and it is wise to refresh or indeed to learn the use of rehabilitative techniques and a wide range of equipment in a local department. The clinical examination vivas are not confined to factual matters of the case in hand and a particular diagnosis frequently leads on directly to a discussion of general principles and practice.

Long case

Arrive in good time at your allotted hospital. It is preferable to bring your own equipment, stethoscope and ophthalmoscope with which you are familiar.

On arrival you will be presented with an examiners' sheet for the long case and one for the short cases. Fill in your name and examination number. You will be asked to hand the relevant sheet to each of the two pairs of examiners, one pair for the long case the other pair for the short cases.

You will be given 45 minutes with your allotted long case to take a full history and to make a physical examination, excluding any invasive procedures. The patient will normally be in a stable condition but may have overt signs of a variety of conditions. There may be communication difficulties as this is not uncommon in elderly patients, and skill and acumen may be needed to obtain a history. Increasingly, carers may be in attendance and if present full use should be made of their help. Failure to do so is heavily penalized. When possible, patients with psychiatric problems are used as long cases (and may also be used as short cases) and candidates should be alert to this and to the psychiatric aspects of patients with primarily physical illness. Lastly, never forget to ask the patient to walk if at all possible. Much can be learned from the observation of gait or its lack or by observing difficulty in rising or moving in bed.

At the end of the 45 minutes you will be escorted to the relevant pair of examiners for a *viva voce* examination, lasting 30 minutes. During this you will be invited to describe the history and your examination findings, your diagnostic conclusions and your suggested plan of management.

The discussion is frequently not confined to the patient under immediate consideration but may lead on to connected matters. Thus a finding of atrial fibrillation may invite discussion of the indications for anticoagulant therapy and by what agents, both in the individual patient and in a population context. Equally the discussion could revolve around both the immediate treatment of the arrhythmia and the place of chemical and electrical attempts at reversal, again both in the individual patient and in the wider policy context. Specific details of, for instance DC conversion, would not be essential, though welcome if known, but the choice of elderly patients seen in general practice for referral to a cardiologist would be very important.

Normal practice is for one of the examiners to lead the discussion for about half the *viva voce* then to hand over to their colleague, who may well embark on a different line of questioning.

So far as possible, the candidate will be taken back to the patient, and carer if present, towards the end of the *viva voce* period in order that the examiners may observe the degree of rapport which has been established with the patient and/or the carer, and to observe the examination technique in the elicitation of physical signs.

After the viva there is a five-minute pause before candidates are introduced to the second pair of examiners for the short cases.

Short cases

The approach to patients acting as short cases is rather different to that applicable to the long case.

Candidates are not left alone with the patient and their approach and attitude to and their physical examination of patients are continually assessed. Second, a complete physical examination is not needed but the elucidation of specific diagnostic points at the examiner's request is required. It is essential to be sure that the request has been fully understood. If in doubt ask. Some examiners can be rather oblique in their approach.

What is being looked for is your approach to the patient: self introduction, common politeness; the accurate assessment of physical signs, in a kindly and thoughtful fashion; a sensible appraisal of the problem and a logical approach to its solution and management. As in the long case, simple diagnosis alone is insufficient, an ability to discuss wider issues and to put them in context is essential. Minutiae are not required.

In addition to patient-based problems you may also be shown videos, usually short, demonstrating such things as abnormal gait, speech difficulties, Parkinson's disease before and after treatment, etc. Again the identification of the particular abnormality is usually a prelude to a wider discussion of treatment and management. The exact diagnosis may be less important than an apposite differential diagnosis from what you observe.

The third group of problems encountered during the short-cases examination is apparatus used by physiotherapists and occupational therapists (a visit to the relevant departments in your own locality before the clinicals is time well spent); a selection of catheters and other devices used in the management of incontinence and occasionally simply laboratory reports, X-rays and ECGs. As always, the standard is that of good quality general practice. In the case of an ECG for instance the recognition of complete heart block, though not difficult, is less important than demonstrating that you realize the possibility of its presence in a patient with vague symptoms and the need for referral for a pacemaker, regardless of chronological age.

The last group of problems commonly met is that of projected slides. These can cover a very wide range of conditions. 'Barn door' diagnoses, e.g. Paget's disease, again are the prelude to discussion of the management of the condition portrayed, in the context of elderly people. Another common condition, steroid-induced Cushing's syndrome, though usually less florid, might lead to a consideration of the range of indications for steroid therapy in elderly people, as well as the common side-effects and might well result in discussion of the management of spinal osteoporosis.

A rather more difficult pair of contrasting spinal X-rays, osteosclerotic and osteoblastic secondaries from carcinoma of the prostrate, could lead to consideration of the differential diagnosis, with a discussion of the various subjects arising, or if the correct diagnosis is arrived at, discussion of the presentation, diagnosis and management of prostatic carcinoma.

Urine rash might cause difficulty initially but leads to discussion of incontinence, the promotion of continence and the prevention of pressure sores.

It is essential to have the capacity to perform an accurate clinical examination and to draw correct conclusions from it, or from associated material, to a standard which demonstrates special interest and ability in the care of elderly people.

However, neither part of the clinical examination is dependent solely on arriving at a correct 'spot' diagnosis. It is the wider knowledge base of the candidate which is also being assessed and particularly the ability to solve problems in a logical fashion and to suggest a sensible plan of management in the overall context in which elderly patients are found.

Marking system

The examination system is carefully arranged to be as fair as possible by ensuring that each candidate is assessed by three pairs of examiners. One pair marks the papers independently of each

Key points

Examination – introduction

- High standard
- Wide syllabus
- Wide potential candidature
- Encapsulates current body of knowledge
- Provides benchmark of expertise for purchasers
- Raises standards of care in general practice
- Aids effectiveness and efficiency in hospital departments

Entry qualifications

- Early in career
- General practice vocational training scheme
- Established GPs
- Potential specialists especially in psychiatry of old age

Preparation

- Read syllabus
  - demographic and social factors
  - clinical aspects of old age
  - administrative aspects of services
- Papers
  - weak areas asked more frequently
- Clinicals
  - current clinical experience with elderly patients

Examination

- Three parts
  - papers
  - long case
  - short cases
- Equal marks between parts
- The papers
  - note currently popular subjects
  - read widely
- Long case
  - good rapport
  - accurate clinical assessment
  - be prepared to discuss wider implications
- Short cases
  - patients, videos, apparatus, slides
  - accuracy in physical signs and diagnosis
  - ability to solve problems
  - appreciation of broader significance

other, the second pair conducts the long case and the third the short cases. All meet together to arrive at a final assessment at the time of the clinical examination.

A degree of compensation is possible between the papers and the clinicals and between the long and short cases in the case of failure of one part, but requires a higher mark overall than a simple pass in all three parts.

Candidates who fail can ask for counselling through the College and this advice is based on the notes made at the time by the examiners. In the case of a particularly bad fail a candidate may be referred for a year. Only four attempts at the diploma are allowed.

Conclusion

Any postgraduate diploma is only earned by the demonstration of particular interest, knowledge, skill and aptitude in the subject. This is equally true of the Diploma in Geriatric Medicine whose remit is very wide covering the whole field of the care of elderly people both individually and in a population context. It is the benchmark of the current state of knowledge in the subject of the management of the elderly at primary care level.

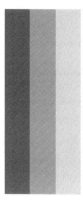

CHAPTER 18

The carer's perspective

Jill Pitkeathley and Carolyn Syverson

For carers, community care has always existed. They were doing it. Most care in the community is provided by so-called 'informal carers' i.e. relatives, neighbours or friends. This is quite significant considering the numbers of people involved. One out of every seven adults cares for a relative or friend who is elderly, ill or disabled. Most carers are between 45 and 64 years of age and most of the people being cared for are over 65.[1] Older carers are more likely to spend long hours caring; some 45% of people caring more than 50 hours a week are over pensionable age.

Who cares?

Being a carer is not unusual. Practically everyone can think of someone in their family or among their friends who is, or at some time was, responsible for the regular care of a mother, father, husband, daughter or friend. It seems a natural thing to do; just one of the potential responsibilities of a normal relationship. This is one reason why many people, including carers themselves, do not recognize carers as a specific group. Because unpaid carers are by definition 'informal' they have not traditionally been seen as having particular needs or rights. For far too long the presence of a carer in a household was the signal for service deliverers to breathe a sigh of relief and withdraw, rather than expand service

provision. It was hoped new community care legislation would do something to change this.

Community care for the carer?

Carers were promised a great deal when the community care changes came into full effect on 1 April 1993. In theory, community care is good for carers and this certainly was intended. However, a reduction in institutional care, the increasing age of the population and constraints on public spending have meant that more and more carers find that services are simply not available when the need arises and they are still expected to cope with very little support. Most carers who have had their needs as carers assessed have found community care plans disappointing, the quality of consultation patchy and a general absence of a realistic planning strategy.[2] The majority of carers have noticed little if any improvement as a result of the 1993 community care changes and many believe services have actually deteriorated and/or become more expensive.[3]

In reality, community care has achieved only limited success in helping carers. There are many reasons for this and many theories about how to make it more effective.

Because much of the practical help in the home has been developed to suit the needs of people living alone, it is often inappropriate for the needs of carers. This is particularly significant for older carers who may be frail or ill themselves. Policy-makers may have to face difficult decisions about whether existing services can be adapted in a way which will make them suitable for carers, or whether they will have to provide something completely new. It is vital that carers' needs for practical help should be regularly reviewed and this help must always be offered with real regard to the particular circumstances of the carer and of the person they look after. It is often a salutary lesson for service providers in both the voluntary and statutory sector, to be reminded that carers neither know, nor care, which agency provides a service, as long as the service:

- meets their particular needs

- is appropriate for the person concerned

- is accessible to the person concerned

- does not have to be sought by the carer 'cap in hand'.

The financial effects of providing care can be devastating. Extra heating, washing, special food and equipment, transport and substitute care all put a huge strain on household budgets. A cost much less easy to quantify is the loss of income for a carer who has had to give up work – a cost that relates not only to the current situation, but also to the future, since in taking on the supporting role carers may be building up poverty for themselves at a later stage in their lives. So carers need realistic levels of benefits, opportunities to maximize the benefits which currently exist and to be able to continue in paid work or to take up employment wherever possible and appropriate. Older carers may find the provisions they made for their retirement no longer adequate. Invalid care allowance is designed to compensate carers but first-time claimants cannot be over the age of 65. Some older carers use their entire savings in the process of caring – some have even lost their homes.[4]

Practical support and recognition

Relief from caring is vital and because there is a wide variety of need there must be a wide variety of provision. Some carers want respite care provided in the home, others want it provided in some kind of residential setting or a mixture of both. It should be borne in mind that time off should not always mean that the carer has to leave the house – the value of privacy in one's own home is too easy to forget. Respite should not be considered a privilege but an integral part of community care planning.

Carers need access to a wide range of information. They need to know about services available in their area, about benefits to which they are entitled, about what being a carer means, about changes in legislation which affect them and where appropriate, as much information as possible about the condition and treatment of the person for whom they are caring. Responsibility for the dissemination of information to carers has never been clearly defined.

The Carers (Recognition and Services) Act, 1 April 1996, goes some way to addressing these needs. The first and most important effect is that it formalizes the existence of carers in law and enjoins this recognition on health and social services. It requires social services to assess their needs along with those of the person in their care upon request. Local authorities are required to take the results of a carer's assessment into account when making decisions about services to be provided for the person cared for and ensure that the user and carer should both be as involved as possible in discussions about the results of assessments and proposed care plans. Consultation should be clearly defined and have minimum standards. The 1996/97 NHS Priorities and Planning Guidance advises a '... greater voice and influence to users of NHS Services and their carers in their own care, the development and definition of standards set for NHS services locally and the development of NHS policy both locally and nationally'. This could influence professional attitudes in practice by making it part of the normal process of needs assessment.

Changing attitudes

This means that professionals need to make some changes in their own attitude to carers. Attitude is a far bigger constraint on progress than restricted resources. At present, too many people hold stereotypical images of what carers are like. Most commonly they are seen as either a martyr or a victim. If the former they are someone giving up their freedom in order to care for someone else. Professionals sometimes find themselves feeling so guilty about them that this guilt gets in the way of proper communication. As one nurse once put it 'I don't ask carers too much about their situations because I'm afraid of what the answers might be'. Similarly, if carers are seen as victims, they are then treated as people who 'need to be needed' and have trapped themselves into the caring relationship out of personal weakness. Realistic views of carers and realistic ways of meeting carers' needs must therefore become integrated into professional thinking. Only then can realistic methods of service provision be established.

Clearly, more resources are an issue but it is not as simple as that. More money would not necessarily make it right, because above all attitudes have to change. To think of carers and elderly people as partners in planning and providing services, rather than as recipients, can be difficult for people who have been trained to think of themselves as providers. Offering choice however, can seem threatening and may lead the professional to ask questions which they will be able to answer, rather than the questions which should be asked. This attitude is frustrating yet understandable. However most carers do not want to stop caring, nor do they want a great deal of interference in their lives; a little more support is usually all they need.

Planning with carers

How do you make it possible for carers to participate in the planning processes? Obvious steps include ensuring they know about the consultation by using the media and public relations department, adapting planning structures so that they can participate; and offering training to carers and professionals.

The difficulties of changing long-held attitudes and of trying to balance the needs of the carer and of the person cared for should be acknowledged and openly discussed and negotiated. Elderly people and their carers are not used to being consulted in this way and most find it difficult to cope with the complicated systems and feel powerless in the face of what they feel is superior knowledge. As one carer said, 'It wasn't that they were horrible to me or anything, on the contrary, they couldn't have been nicer. The

doctor got up and brought my coffee to me and they kept saying that I was the most important person in the equation and about the package of care they were going to put on for mother. But I don't know what an equation is to be honest, or a package of care come to that. I just didn't feel I could say how frightened I was. It would have sounded so feeble and somehow ungrateful. That's odd really because they all kept saying how grateful they were to me'. The message for professional carers is to communicate simply and clearly with informal carers without being patronizing.

Primary health care

The great majority of carers want help and advice from health professionals. Around 40% of carers see their general practice as the main source of information, help and advice.[5] Most general practitioners (GPs) however, do not agree with this description. They may be sympathetic but do not see what they can provide to someone who is not ill and carers are not a priority within health promotion. General practice is going through major changes as a result of community care legislation, the NHS reforms and the shift from secondary to primary care. It is not surprising that GPs feel they are being asked to provide too much support, too quickly.[6] The reality is that GPs and the primary health care team can provide a great deal which will not necessarily increase demand on time or resources.

Where appropriate, carers need information about the condition of the person for whom they are caring and the treatment they may be receiving. It is not unusual for a carer to feel frightened and unsure about what they are dealing with and whether or not they are being competent and effective. At present, although carers give most of the hands-on-care they are not considered part of the health care team and are frequently left to cope with various stages of illness and drug side-effects with little or no advice, information or reassurance.

General practitioners are seen by carers as the professionals who can make the difference to their lives 'if you've got a good GP, you're made' as one put it. By this carers do not mean that they want a GP who will provide them with endless services, but rather one who will recognize their situation and acknowledge their problems. Above all, they want a GP who will listen. GPs, and primary care workers in general, have a greater part to play in the lives of carers than ever before. The Carers Act recommends social services to provide the environment of communication between providers that community care has so far lacked.

Developing a carers' code

To be effective, those providing community care need to listen to carers so that the provision of services is 'needs led'.

Carers need:

- **Recognition:** Real recognition for who they are and what they do, their expertise and skill, their need for services. Recognition that being a carer does not mean they cease to be a person in their own right.

- **Equity:** Recognition of the needs of carers should not be biased by gender assumptions, cultural differences, age, sexual orientation, race or disability.

- **Information:** A system of clear responsibility needs to be established for signposting carers to information about benefits entitlement, medical conditions, treatments and their side-effects, support groups, etc. Service providing agencies should work in coordination and communicate effectively with each other. Good communication with the carer is also vital.

- **Consultation:** Carers should be involved in consultation through representation and direct participation.

- **Practical support:** Assessment procedures should be speedy, well thought out and accessible. Flexible carer-focused services should be developed.

- **Financial support:** Only about 17.5% of full-time carers receive Invalid Care Allowance, which is only available to first-time claimants under 65. Most carers live on fixed incomes with virtually no hope of continuing or taking up employment. Many carers are asked to pay for services being given to the person for whom they are caring. Carers should be helped to access benefits, assistance if they want to work outside the home and a voice in policy regarding charges.

- **The right to say 'no more':** Caring is a relationship, and in any relationship there is change. Sometimes carers become physically or mentally exhausted to the point that they can no longer cope with the responsibility. No one should be forced to be a carer, nor should they be forced to continue if they feel they cannot.

Conclusion

The value of carers to the community is virtually incalculable. Some estimate that the care they provide saves providers as much as £36 billion each year. But it is only relatively recently that the 6.9 million people caring for family and friends have been at least partially recognized. Responsibility for implementing community care needs to be better defined in practice. Professionals need to be committed to truly effective consultation and communication. They need to plan more strategically and be more realistic and flexible in organizing services to support carers. To do this they above all need to give the provision for carers, in concept and reality, the importance it deserves.

References

1 Warner N (1994) *Just a Fairy Tale.* Carers National Association, London.
2 Hudson B (1995) Could do better. *Health Service Journal* **105**:30–1.
3 Warner N (1995) *Better Tomorrow's.* Carers National Association, London.
4 Alison V and Wright F (1990) *Still Caring.* The Spastics Society and the final report of the Carnegie Inquiry into the Third Age.
5 Yee L and Blunden R (1995) *General Practice and Carers: Scope for change?* King's Fund Centre, London.
6 Duggan M (1995) *Primary Health Care – A Prognosis.* Institute for Public Policy Research, London.

Further reading

BMA (1995) *Taking Care of the Carers.* Report. February. BMA, London.
CNA, Speak Up, Speak Out, 1992. London.

Eagles JM, Craig A, Rawlinson F *et al.* (1987) The psychological well-being of supporters of the demented elderly. *Br J Psychiatry* **150**:293–8.

Livingston G, Manela MM and Katona C (1996) Psychiatric morbidity in carers of elderly people living at home. *BMJ* **312**:153–6.

O'Connor DW, Pollitt PA, Roth R *et al.* (1990) Problems reported by relatives in a community study of dementia. *Br J Psychiatry* **156**:835–41.

Appendix 1:

The Bicester system of screening for the elderly

Summary of 'screening' programme

1 Register of patients – this was completed for patients aged over 75 years, stratified and called up for review in the following sequence:

   i) patients known to be significantly 'at risk' a) over 85 years b) 75–84 years

   ii) patients not significantly 'at risk' a) over 85 years b) 75–84 years

2 Letter sent by their GP to each patient enclosing a health questionnaire (Form A) and advising the patient that a volunteer visitor (VV) would be calling on behalf of the practice to ask some questions about their quality of life (Form B). The patient was advised that this would help the practice to organize their care more effectively. Patients were given the opportunity to refuse the service. The visitors had to produce a 'passport' before being admitted to the patients' homes – signed authorization by the GP with the visitor's picture on it. Form B was meant to identify and scale problems and patients were held to be vulnerable if below the •••••••• lines. VVs were given special training on sensitive subjects, such as urinary and bowel problems or financial status.

The completed health questionnaire could be sent by post to the health centre or given to the visitor in a sealed envelope. A surprising number of the patients however, especially if living alone, asked the visitor for help in completing the questionnaire even on the most intimate and personal of topics.

3 Two weeks later the patients – if fit enough – were called to a 'seniors' clinic at the health centre for a physical assessment of health and function and a briefing on health education by the nurse or health visitor (Form C) and doctor. Sometimes this review had to be done at home because the patient was unfit to come to the surgery or the home environment needed to be assessed.

4 A problem profile was then compiled based on all these findings and with particular emphasis on functional status (Form D) – the Barthel Index was completed when patients were only disabled.

5 Patient adaptation to their problems was then assessed.

6 Current therapy was carefully reviewed.

7 A management plan was then made tailored to the patient's needs.

8 The patient's risk status was then estimated.

9 Finally the date of the next review was then recorded.

Volunteer visitors' role

The completion of Form B can be done by the practice nurse or health visitor if they have time. However, we chose intelligent, recently retired lay people as they had more time available and the completion of this form took 30–45 minutes in each case. These workers were given training in the use of the form with particular emphasis on sensitive matters, such as asking about financial status. They also had to give signed undertakings about the confidentiality of information involved.

Nurse's role

The nurse will see the patient first, review the health questionnaire, socio-economic and functional position, check the height, weight, BP, urine, sight and hearing after which he or she will make a general report using the check-list on the form as an aide memoire. This is not a tick-off check-list.

Doctor's role

1 The doctor must first review the problems already identified in:

a) the questionnaire on socio-economic and functional problems
b) the health questionnaire
c) the nursing assessment.

2 Focused physical assessment as seems indicated by the above findings – also the institution of appropriate investigations.

3 Review of therapy to ensure that it remains currently appropriate:

– review prescription card
– medicine memory card.

4 Review of the need for aids.

5 *Retirement pension*: a) based on your own contribution record and b) based on your partner's contribution record if you are a married woman or your partner has died.

Income support: can top up income to a set level which depends upon age and personal circumstances.

Social fund: provides help to those on income support who need a one-off sum to meet expenses of any kind – paid either as a grant or a loan.

Housing benefit: for those on low-income living in rented accommodation.

Council tax benefit: means-tested for those on a low income.

Attendance allowance: for those needing help with personal care or supervision from another person because of physical or mental disability.

Prescription charges: free to those over pension age (65 for men, 60 for women).

6 Assessment of need under provisions of NHS and Community Care Act:

– help with personal care – care assistant or similar worker
– meals on wheels
– help with domestic tasks usually only available if a care package is in place
– alarms
– luncheon clubs
– day centres
– day care
– respite care
– laundry services – if available, it will normally be run by social services and district health authority
– other services – detail.

7 Listing of those problems likely to affect the well being and enjoyment of day-to-day life (this information is based on the information in forms A, B and C and is recorded in form D):

– socio-economic
– functional
– psychological
– medical.

8 The patient's adaptation to these problems is then assessed.

9 Carer's status – the quality of this support is surveyed for its effectiveness and evidence of carer stress.

10 Priorities of need can then be established and an appropriate programme of care developed for each patient.

11 Referral to other agencies is then considered:

- hospital specialist
- nurse/care assistant

- chiropodist
- occupational therapist
- physiotherapist
- health visitor/
  bath attendant

- deaf visitor
- home help
  supervisor
- Red Cross
- housing officer
- volunteer worker
- warden sheltered
  accommodation

- dentist
- social worker
- optician
- blind visitor
- speech therapist

- floating bed
- family support
- hairdresser
- library

12 Finally, the patient is given a risk rating and a decision is taken on the review interval.

It was found that when the roles of the volunteer visitors, nurse and GP were carefully systematized results were much better than using an informal approach.

The health education component of the nurses' work proved particularly important.

FORM A

	Assessment of the Elderly Basic Health Questionnaire	
Name: Address: D.O.B.		Date:

		Yes	Please give details

1   *Compared with two years ago:*

Is your sight poorer?   ❏

Is your hearing poorer?   ❏

If so, do you have a hearing aid?   ❏

Do you feel more tired?   ❏

Has your weight changed?   ❏

Are you more breathless?   ❏

Do you pass water more often?   ❏
– especially at night?

Can you move about as freely?   ❏

Is your memory poorer:
– for recent events?   ❏
– for events long ago?   ❏

Is your concentration poorer?   ❏

Is your appetite poor?   ❏

Do you often feel low in spirits?   ❏

Are you more troubled by anxiety?   ❏

Do you have difficulty regularly in getting off   ❏
    to sleep or do you often wake early in the morning?

	Yes	Please give details
2 *Do you have any of the following:*		
dizzy spells	❏	
blackouts	❏	
falls	❏	
fits	❏	
pains in:		
head	❏	
chest	❏	
abdomen	❏	
legs on walking	❏	
elsewhere	❏	
breathlessness	❏	
persistent cough	❏	
dental problems – painful or carious teeth, ill-fitting dentures, etc.	❏	
difficulty in swallowing	❏	
indigestion	❏	
constipation or diarrhoea	❏	
bed wetting (urine)/soiling (motion)	❏	
swollen ankles	❏	
foot problems, e.g. corns or bunions affecting walking	❏	
pain or swelling of joints	❏	
3 Can you move about as well as 12 months ago?	❏	
4 Have you been in hospital in the past year?	❏	
5 Have you any other health problems?	❏	

FORM B

Assessment of the Elderly
Health Questionnaire

Name:
Address:
D.O.B.   Date:

A. SOCIO-ECONOMIC PROBLEMS

1   Day-to-day support
i.   Lives with spouse
ii.   Lives with children
iii. Lives with other relatives
iv. Lives with friends

****

v.   Lives alone with periodic outside
      support
vi. Lives alone without support

___

2   Illness support
      When confined to bed the patient has:
i. · Full support
ii.   Day-time support only

****

iii. Uncertain support
iv. No support

___

3   Accommodation A-Good; B-Fair; C-Poor
      Structural state
      Heating
      Running H & C
      Toilet facilities
      Lighting
      Decoration

      Rating of structure and facilities:
i.   Excellent
ii.   Good
iii. Fair

****

iv. Poor
v.   Unacceptable

Suitability of accommodation:
i.   Good
ii.   Fair

****

iii. Poor

___

4   Social contact
      Relatives, friends or neighbours seen:
i.   Daily
ii.   Two/Three times a week
iii. Weekly

****

iv. Sporadically
v.   Rarely

___

5   Economic status
i.   Satisfactory
ii.   Borderline

****

iii. Inadequate

___

6   Recent bereavement
      During the past year patient has lost:
i.   Nobody
ii.   A close friend, in-law, or relative
      outside the immediate family
iii. Parent
iv. A husband, wife or child

___

7   Loneliness
      The patient feels lonely:
i.   Never
ii.   Occasionally

****

iii. Often
iv. Almost all the time

8   Accident risk
i.   Minimal
ii. Average

9   Other problems
a)   Infirm partner   YES/NO
b)   Frustration   YES/NO
c)   Boredom   YES/NO
d)   Lack of role/purpose   YES/NO

10 Need for
a)   Meals on wheels
b)   Transport
c)   Help with shopping
d)   Home visiting
e)   Day centre
f)   Luncheon club
g)   Other (please state)

B.   PROBLEMS OF DISABILITY

1   Mobility
i.   Fully mobile
ii. Moderate impairment of mobility
****
iii. Marked limitation of mobility
     (no aid or assistance)
iv. Mobile only with aid
v.   Mobile only with assistance
     (iii, iv and v usually housebound)
vi. Bed or chair fast

2   Continence
i.   Fully continent
ii. Occasional accident due to restricted
     mobility of stress incontinence
****
iii. Nocturnal incontinence of urine
iv. Urinary incontinence day and night
v.   Double incontinence

3   Domestic care
     Cooking
i.   Able to prepare all meals
ii. Able to prepare some food only
iii. Unable to prepare food/meals at all
     Housework
i.   Able to do all own housework
ii. Requires assistance with housework
iii. Requires full-time help

Shopping
i.   Able to do all own shopping
ii. Requires assistance with shopping
iii. Unable to do any shopping
     Rating
i.   Scores 1 in all indices
ii. Scores 2 on no more than one index
iii. Scores 2 on more than one index
iv. Scores 3 on two or three indices

4   Nutrition
i.   Adequate
ii. Borderline
****
iii. Unsatisfactory

5   Self-care
     Dressing
i.   Independent
ii. Requires assistance with shoes and
     socks only
iii. Able to assist in dressing
iv. Unable to assist in dressing
     Feeding
i.   Independent
ii. Requires assistance with cutting up
     food only
iii. Able to assist in feeding
iv. Unable to assist in feeding
     Toilet
i.   Independent day and night
ii. Requires assistance at night only
iii. Requires assistance day and night but
     remains continent
iv. Incontinent despite assistance
     Rating
i.   Fully independent – scores 1 in each
ii. Minor disability – scores 2 in each
     except dressing, where they may score 2
****
iii. Partial independence – scores 2 or 3 on
     feeding and/or toilet or 3 on dressing
iv. Dependent – scores 4 on at least one
     index
v.   Wholly dependent – scores 4 on two
     or three indices

6   Transferring
i.   Independent
****
ii. Needs help

7   Other problems

FORM C

	Assessment of the Elderly Nursing Report
Name: Address: D.O.B.	Date:

Review health questionnaire and, using the following check-list, report your findings on the patient's health and functional status:

appearance   _____

speech   _____

behaviour   _____

attitude   _____

posture   _____

gait   _____

mentation   _____

emotional state   _____

? pallor   _____

teeth   _____

tremor (nature)   _____

breathlessness   _____

weakness or paralysis   _____

? arthritis   _____

swollen ankles   _____

ulcers leg/feet   _____

corns/bunions, etc.   _____

The nurse is asked to give her appreciation of the older person's state of health and function with particular relevance to the factors listed to help her. This is **not** simply a check-list and the nurse may also report on other factors.

Sensory impairment:

a.   *Sight*

Has the patient any problems:

i.   Watching TV   ❏

ii.   Reading newspapers   ❏

iii.   Other circumstances   ❏

Snellen Test Type:

	R	L
Near		
Distant		

b.   *Hearing*

Are the ears clear of wax or debris?   ❏

Does the patient have difficulty with:

i.   Ordinary conversation   ❏

ii.   Conversation   ❏

iii.   Listening to TV   ❏

iv.   On the telephone   ❏

v.   In other circumstances   ❏

Audiometry

BP   *Weight*   *Urine*

Health Education – Nutrition

Exercise

Warmth

Home safety

Security

Disability benefits

Social contacts

General information

The nurse will also do a Mini-Mental State examination (see Chapter 4) in cases where it is thought appropriate.

FORM D

Assessment of the Elderly
Problem Profile/Action Risk Index

Name:
Address:
D.O.B.

Date:

Current medical disorders (acute)	Previous medical history (inactive)
1 2 3 4 5 6 7 8	1 2 3 4 5 6 7 8

Socio-economic and functional status

1 Mobility – normal for age, impaired, needs aids, chairbound 2 Gait 3 Cooking 4 Housework 5 Shopping 6 Transferring 7 Dressing 8 Feeding	9 Tendency to dizzy spells, falls, faints, drop attacks, fits 10 Mental state 11 Continence 12 Speech 13 Sight 14 Hearing 15 Socialization 16 Other

Current therapy

1 2 3 4 5	6 7 8 9 10

Adaptation to problems

a) Very good
b) Good
c) Fair
d) Poor

Special requirements	Drug sensitivities

Supporters		
Name	Address	Relationship
1		
2		
3		
4		

Action

Risk index	
Medical problems	Socio-economic problems
1 Nil	Nil
2 Minor and/or	Minor
3 a) Minor and b) Nil or minor and	Nil or minor
4 Major	Major
5 Dependent	Major
6 Wholly dependent	
Next assessment in	Months/years

The disability form in this system was designed and validated by Professor FI Caird, Emeritus Professor, Department of Geriatric Medicine of Glasgow University. The rest of the system was designed and (where necessary) validated by Alistair Tulloch.

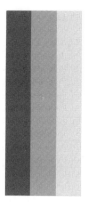

Appendix 2:
McIntosh over 75s assessment questionnaire – data store

NAME: .... CIVIL STATUS: M | S | W | D ADDRESS: .... TELEPHONE: .... TYPE OF HOUSING:	NAME AND RELATIONSHIP OF CARING RELATIVE OR NEXT OF KIN: ADDRESS: .... TELEPHONE:	CODE No: [＿＿＿] DATE OF BIRTH: / / GP: .... HV: .... REPEAT SCRIPT [＿＿＿] CARD NO CAN VISIT SURGERY? Yes ☐ No ☐

SERVICES NEEDED: (R = REQUIRED, P = PROVIDED, D = DISCONTINUED, Ref = REFUSED)

DATE											
CHIROPODY											
DAY HOSPITAL											
DENTAL CARE											
OPTICIAN											
AUDIOMETRY											
DISTRICT NURSE											
HEALTH VISITOR											
SOCIAL WORKER											
HOME HELP											
HOSPITAL											
RE-HOUSING											
RESPITE CARE											
MEALS ON WHEELS											
OCCUPATIONAL THERAPIST											
OTHERS											

ACTIVITIES OF DAILY LIVING:

DATE											
SCORE – HOUSEHOLD											
0 Fully independent											
1 Friend or relative lives with them											
2 Friend or relative visits regularly											
3 Dependent on social services											
4 Dependent on community nurses etc.											
5 Combination											
Sub-totals											
BEREAVEMENT OF SPOUSE OR SIBLING											
0 None											
3 Less than 2 years											
5 Less than 6 months											
Sub-totals											
SCORE – HOUSING											
0 No problems											
1 Too big											
2 Too many stairs											
4 Damp or poor conditions of housing											
5 Multiple housing problems											
Sub-totals											
WARMTH											
0 Adequate											
3 Barely adequate											
5 Inadequate											
Sub-totals											
MOBILITY											
0 Full mobility											
2 Mobile with aids											
4 Housebound											
5 Bed or chairbound											
Sub-totals											

/continued …

ACTIVITIES OF DAILY LIVING: ... (continued)

DATE											
CONTINENCE											
0 Fully continent											
2 Stress incontinence or urgency											
4 Day/night incontinence											
5 Incontinent of urine and faeces											
Sub-totals											
VISION											
0 Satisfactory											
1 Uses vision aid											
3 Partially sighted											
5 Blind											
Sub-totals											
HEARING											
0 No noticeable loss											
1 Satisfactory with hearing aid											
3 Unsatisfactory with/without aid											
5 Total deafness											
Sub-totals											
HYGIENE											
0 Satisfactory											
1 Satisfactory with aids											
3 Bath or shower with assistance											
4 Dirty and unkempt											
Sub-totals											
DIET											
0 Satisfactory											
1 Satisfactory with supplied meals											
3 Deficient											
Sub-totals											

/continued ...

ACTIVITIES OF DAILY LIVING: ... (continued)

DATE												
SCORE – WEIGHT												
0 Normal												
2 Moderately obese												
4 Underweight/obese												
5 Very underweight/very obese												
Sub-totals												
SLEEP												
0 Sleeps well without sedation												
2 Disturbed sleep												
3 Sleeps well with sedation												
Sub-totals												
EMOTIONAL ASSESSMENT												
0 No problems												
2 Discontented												
4 Very unhappy												
Sub-totals												

COMMENTS:

MEDICAL ASSESSMENT: (At each assessment score: 0 = no symptoms to 6 = severe symptoms)
Risk: H = High, M = Medium, L = Low

DATE											
1 CARDIOVASCULAR											
2 ENDOCRINE											
3 GASTROINTESTINAL											
4 GENITOURINARY											
5 LOCOMOTOR											
6 MEMORY LOSS											
7 NERVOUS SYSTEM											
8 PSYCHIATRIC											
9 RESPIRATORY											
10 SKIN											
SCORE TOTALS											
MEDICAL											
DAILY LIVING											
CUMULATIVE SCORE											
WEIGHT											
BP											

MENTAL STATUS:

INSTRUCTIONS: Ask questions 1–10 in this list and record all errors.
Ask question 4A only if the patient does not have a telephone.
Record the total number of errors based on 10 questions.
Fully date and sign each entry.

DATE											
1 What is the date today? (d-m-y)											
2 What day of the week is it?											
3 What is the name of this place?											
4 What is your telephone number?											
4A What is your street address? (Ask only if no telephone)											
5 How old are you?											
6 When were you born? (d-m-y)											
7 Who is the Prime Minister now?											
8 Who was the previous Prime Minister?											
9 What was your mother's maiden name?											
10 Take 3 away from 20 and keep taking 3 from each new number you get, all the way down											
TOTAL ERRORS											
Administered by:											

RESULTS:

0–2 errors, intact intellectual function
3–4 errors, mild intellectual impairment
5–7 errors, moderate intellectual impairment
8–10 errors, severe intellectual impairment

MEDICATION/MEDICAL NEEDS:

DATE	PRODUCT	DOSE	NOTES

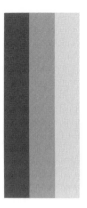

Appendix 3:
Phoenix Surgery Anticipatory Care Model for people over the age of 75 years in Cirencester

Introduction

The present model has evolved over ten years. In 1986, Phoenix services for children were well established with a full-time health visitor supporting 400 children and families under five years of age. A formal system for identification of unmet need for elderly people had not developed and yet in Gloucestershire at that time over 60% of bed days were occupied by people over 75 years of age – 6% of the population.

We now provide primary care to about 10 000 people, with six partners working from a central surgery and three branch surgeries all linked by land-lines and using EMIS computer support. We care for 640 people over 75 years of age. All primary care staff, including community nurses and health visitors, have recently moved to the central surgery site. Each partner maintains a personal list and has a 'special' interest, usually working with Cirencester subdistrict hospital.

Supported by experience as acting consultant geriatrician and hospital practitioner in Cirencester, David Beales thought that the problems experienced by the elderly often centred on practical and functional difficulties, accompanied by feelings of social isolation and disengagement rather than problems solely associated with health. These were already known and largely catered for by existing medical services. A combination of medical, psychological, functional and social/spiritual not unusually led to the

'breakdown' and sometimes unnecessary hospital admission.

Evolution of present working practice

The development of the present working practice evolved from a research project in which trained volunteer visitors, with health visitor support, were able to select and target focused assessment by the health visitor and other professional workers as well as provide social support in a cost-effective way.[1] The finding in this study and in subsequent years that over 50% of people with an average age of 80 years of age had low disability and did not require long-term follow-up or annual review then prompted the introduction of a two-phase screening programme using a well-validated postal questionnaire.[2] This had been piloted in general practice and had not only identified unmet need in 50% of a previously 'unscreened' population but had, following its introduction, significantly reduced hospital admission and institutional care compared with the control group studied.

This 'Cardiff questionnaire' is now used, following further piloting, to detect people with a wide variety of self-perceived problems. The questionnaire is seen by the health visitor who

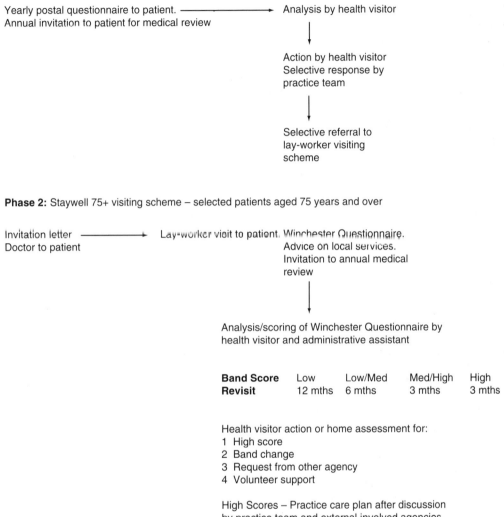

Phase 1: Postal questionnaire system – patients aged 75 years and over – Phoenix Surgery

Yearly postal questionnaire to patient. ⟶ Analysis by health visitor
Annual invitation to patient for medical review

Action by health visitor
Selective response by
practice team

Selective referral to
lay-worker visiting
scheme

Phase 2: Staywell 75+ visiting scheme – selected patients aged 75 years and over

Invitation letter ⟶ Lay-worker visit to patient. Winchester Questionnaire.
Doctor to patient   Advice on local services.
                                          Invitation to annual medical
                                          review

Analysis/scoring of Winchester Questionnaire by
health visitor and administrative assistant

Band Score	Low	Low/Med	Med/High	High
Revisit	12 mths	6 mths	3 mths	3 mths

Health visitor action or home assessment for:
1 High score
2 Band change
3 Request from other agency
4 Volunteer support

High Scores – Practice care plan after discussion
by practice team and external involved agencies.
Coordination and review by key worker

Figure 1 Revisiting schedule dependent on disability score

in conjunction with the clinical notes, and discussion with primary care team members decides on appropriate action. Requests for information only are telephoned to the patient directly by the administrative assistant who follows up non-responders. They often simply need a reminder to complete and return the questionnaire. A 90% response rate was achieved in the initial pilot. After discussion of the findings those who have continuing health or social problems are invited to enter the Staywell surveillance system. These people are then followed up by the trained volunteer visitors who complete the Winchester Disability Questionnaire. They then follow a structured revisiting schedule depending on the disability score (see Figure 1).

The doctors choose to carry out a separate annual elderly medical review to all patients over the age of 75 years who take up the invitation to attend as well as much lengthier and detailed reviews for those with high disability or on multiple medication. This policy is under review.

The Staywell 75+ team consists of a health visitor employed by the practice for 20 hours a week with 70% reimbursement.[3] A supporting doctor represents the partnership. An administrative assistant is employed for nine hours a week, with 70% reimbursement and 24 lay workers divided into two groups, with team leaders, who are trained and then meet regularly with the health visitor who organizes monthly group discussions with outside agencies. The volunteer expenses – about £800 a year are provided from the Phoenix Surgery Charitable Trust. Insurance for volunteers is provided through the local volunteer bureau which assists with recruitment and external support. A quarterly review meeting of the team including the team leaders for the layworkers meets to review, clarify aims and objectives and to set future policy. Recruitment of lay workers is increasingly from within the practice and an introductory weekly training of six sessions is held in the autumn. The lay workers stay on average for three years.

The administrative assistant enters data and prompts the lay workers on the follow-up dates. The doctors add the record of their elderly medical review on the computer template. An audit cycle and review of the whole system is readily available.

Future possibilities

The practice is now committed, with the aid of development grants, to identify the needs of all disabled patients, and assess patient and carer support requirements through the development of a shared computer record used by all members of the practice. Suitable assessment measures that can be integrated into normal practice routine will be agreed before introduction. This information will allow the practice to define need and to purchase and provide appropriate care.

Key points

- A structured model for the anticipatory care of elderly people is described. Clear roles and responsibilities have evolved with the development of a working practice which has allowed in the last ten years more effective multi-disciplinary working and anticipatory care

- The system as described has promoted the focused deployment of scarce professional practice resources

- The cost has been modest

- The volunteers act as the extended arm of community care

References

1 Beales D and Hicks E (1988) Volunteers help to detect unreported problems in the elderly. *The Practitioner* **232**:478–82.

2 Pathy MS, Bayer A, Harding K *et al.* (1992) Randomised trial of case finding and surveillance of elderly people at home. *Lancet* **340**: 890–3.

3 Beales D and Hicks E (1993) *Staywell 75+: preventive home visits to people aged 75 and over with trained volunteers from within a group general practice.* Phoenix Surgery, Cirencester.

Further reading

Beales D (1982) A new form of community hospital service for the elderly. *BMJ* **284**:840–8.

Carpenter GI and Demopoulos GR (1990) Screening the elderly in the community: controlled trial of dependency surveillance using a questionnaire administered by volunteers. *BMJ* **300**:1253–6.

CARDIFF-NEWPORT QUESTIONNAIRE
AMENDED VERSION 1992

Name .... Today's date ....

Address ....

....

....

Date of Birth .... Telephone No ....

General Practitioner ....

Practice Address ....

....

**PLEASE ANSWER EACH QUESTION BY <u>CIRCLING</u> THE
APPROPRIATE NUMBER OR <u>WRITING IN THE SPACE PROVIDED</u>**

---

1 Do you live alone?

Yes	1
No	2

If NO, who else lives in the household with you?

....

....

---

2 How has your health been over the past month?

Very good	1
Good	2
Poor	3
Very poor	4

---

3 During the past month, how many days have you been ill at all?

None	1
1 to 7 days	2
8 to 14 days	3
15 days or more	4

Give details ....

....

....

4   Please circle any of the following conditions you
     <u>currently</u> have at this time

1	Heart condition	12	Liver disease
2	Circulation problems	13	Kidney disease
3	High blood pressure	14	Urinary problems
4	Anaemia	15	Parkinson's disease
5	Diabetes	16	Stroke
6	Bronchitis/Emphysema	17	Arthritis
7	Cataracts	18	Foot problems
8	Stomach ulcers	19	Problems with 'nerves'
9	Broken bones	20	Skin problems
10	Gall bladder problems	21	Cancer
11	Hernia	22	Other (list) ....

....

....

5   Give details of any medicines you are <u>currently</u> taking

1	Arthritis medication	12	Antibiotics ....
2	Pain killers	13	Thyroid pills ....
3	Sleeping pills	14	Seizure pills ....
4	Allergy pills	15	Chest pain pills ....
5	High blood pressure pills	16	Water pills ....
	....	17	Laxatives ....
6	Pills for diabetes	18	Blood thinning medication ....
7	Heart pills		....
8	Insulin	19	Medication for breathing ....
9	Stomach medicine		....
10	Tranquillizers	20	Circulation pills ....
11	Steroids/cortisone	21	Other (list) ....
	....		....

6   Do you have any problems with medication?

	Yes	1
	No	2

7   Do you have any physical disability that limits your daily activities?

	No, none	1
	Some limitation	2
	Moderate limitation	3
	Severe limitation	4

Give details ....

,,,,,,,,,,,...

....

8   Have you had any falls in the past month?

	No, none	1
	Yes (give details)	2

....

....

9   Have you been more unsteady when walking in the last 3 months?

	Not at all	1
	A little	2
	Quite a bit	3

10   Do you have difficulty getting up from a chair?

	Not at all	1
	A little	2
	Quite a bit	3

and/or Do you have difficulty getting up from bed?

	Not at all	1
	A little	2
	Quite a bit	3

11 Are you able to walk ...		
	Without help	1
	With some help (such as a stick or frame)	2
	With quite a bit of help (such as help from another person)	3
	Cannot walk at all	4
12 Do you have difficulty in getting up and down stairs or steps?		
	No, not at all	1
	A little	2
	Quite a bit	3
	Cannot manage stairs or steps at all	4
13 Are you able to get to places that are <u>not</u> within walking distance ...		
	Without help using bus, taxi, car, etc.	1
	With a little help	2
	With quite a bit of help	3
	Cannot travel even with help (need ambulance)	4
14 Are you able to go shopping for groceries or clothes?		
	By yourself, without help	1
	With a little help	2
	With quite a bit of help	3
	Cannot go shopping at all	4
15 How often do you see your friends or relatives?		
	Often (daily or several times a week)	1
	Occasionally (about once a week)	2
	Infrequently (about once a month)	3
	Rarely or never	4

16 How often have you worked on a hobby or some activity
of interest over the last month?

Often	1
Occasionally	2
Infrequently	3
Not at all	4

17 How often have you attended meetings at associations,
church, pub, get-together, etc. over the past month?

Often (several times a week)	1
Occasionally (weekly)	2
Seldom (once during the month)	3
Never	4

18 Are you able to do most of the chores that need doing
around the house …

Without help, for example cook, garden, houseclean, etc.	1
With a little help	2
With quite a bit of help	3
Cannot do chores at all	4

19 Are you able to take care of your appearance, such as
comb your hair, shave, put on make-up, etc. …

Without help	1
With some help	2
With quite a bit of help	3
Cannot take care of appearance at all	4

20 Are you able to dress yourself …

Without help – for example choosing own clothes, buttoning and zipping them, etc.	1
With a little help	2
With quite a bit of help	3
Cannot manage at all	4

21 Do you have difficulty in passing water (e.g. starting, stopping, a poor stream, or associated discomfort)

Not at all	1
Sometimes	2
Quite often	3
Always	4

22 Can you bath or shower ...

Without help	1
With special devices to help you	2
With someone to help you	3
Cannot have a bath or shower at all (must have bed bath)	4

23 Do you ever have an 'accident' if you are unable to get to a toilet as soon as you need to, or when you are asleep, or if you cough or sneeze?

No, never	1
Only occasionally	2
Quite often	3
Frequently	4
Have catheter/colostomy	5

24 Do you have any significant problems with your eyesight?

No, none	1
Yes (give details)	2

....

....

25 Do you have any significant problems with your hearing?

No, none	1
Yes (give details)	2

....

....

26 Are you able to handle your own money ...

Without help – for example, pay bills, Write your own cheques, etc.	1
With a little help	2
With quite a bit of help	3
Cannot manage money at all	4

27 Do you, or other people, think you are forgetful?

No	1
Yes	2

If <u>YES</u>

a) Has your memory deteriorated
during the past year?

No	1
Yes	2

b) Does your memory interfere with
your everyday life

No	1
Yes	2

28 Are you able to use the telephone ...

Without help, including looking up numbers	1
With a little help	2
With quite a bit of help	3
Unable to use 'phone	4
Do not have access to 'phone	5

29 At present, do you receive any of the services listed?

Home help	1
Meals on wheels	2
Day Centre/Luncheon Club, etc.	3
Day hospital	4
Chiropody	5
Attendance allowance	6
District nurse	7
Any other (give details)	8

....

....

30 Do you feel you would be helped by provision of any of the
    following services?

Home help	1
Meals on wheels	2
Day centre attendance	3
Chiropody	4
Dental care	5
Dietician	6
Hearing aid	7
Optician	8
Housing advice	9
Additional financial help (i.e. rent/ rates rebate, heating benefit, attendance allowance, etc.)	10
Other (explain)	11

....

....

31 Have you been feeling particularly sad or unhappy recently?

No, not at all	1
A little	2
Quite a bit	3
Extremely	4

32 Have you been feeling particularly worried or irritable recently?

No, not at all	1
A little	2
Quite a bit	3
Extremely	4

33 Can you now do all the things that you could do last year?

Yes	1
No	2

If NO, give examples:

....

....

....

34 Is there anything about your health at present
    which is causing you any concern or difficulty?

No	1
Yes	2

If YES, would you give further details:

....

....

....

35 Did you complete this questionnaire ...

By yourself	1
With help (give relationship of person who helped you)	2

....

THANK YOU FOR YOUR CO-OPERATION

To help people say how good or
bad a health state is, we have
drawn a scale (rather like a
thermometer) on which the best
state you can imagine is marked
by 100 and the worse state you
can imagine is marked by 0.
Please mark with a cross on this
scale how good or bad you think
your own health is today.

100 (best imaginable state)

90

80

70

60

50

40

30

20

10

0 (worst imaginable state)

Training Programme for Staywell 75+ Volunteer Visiting Scheme

7 Sessions – 1 hour 30 mins – weekly

Aim of scheme

To promote good health and wellbeing in patients registered with Phoenix Surgery who are 75 years of age and over, with the help of trained volunteer visitors.

Aim of training programme

To extend knowledge of the purpose of the volunteer visiting scheme and the role of the volunteer visitor within the scheme.

Objectives of training programme

After the training programme the visitor should be:

- aware of the role of the volunteer visitor within the scheme

- aware of the relationship between volunteer, client and professional

- able to outline certain circumstances which may lead to stress in an elderly person's life

- able to use some preliminary counselling skills

- able to record information using the specified questionnaire

- able to summon professional help and advice when needed

- able to give some information on state and voluntary help available to the elderly

Winchester Questionnaire

SURNAME: [   ] Forename: Date of birth:

ADDRESS:

NAME OF GP:

Marital Status:	Widowed		Married	Single		Divorced/Separated
Who do you live with?	Alone		Spouse only	Sp + other rel		Other
Type of Residence?	GF Flat	Flat + lift	Bungalow	Whole House	Part House Pt III	R/Home N/Home

How many falls within the <u>last month</u>? [   ]

1	WALKING	Independent	Semi-independent	Housebound can manage stairs	Housebound can't manage stairs	Chairfast or bedfast
2	DRESSING/ UNDRESSING	Independent	Some difficulty	Much difficulty	Manages with help	Needs dressing
3	WASHING	Independent	Some difficulty	Much difficulty	Manages with help	Needs washing
4	BATHING	Independent	Some difficulty	Much difficulty	Manages with help	Needs bathing
5	EATING	Independent normal diet	Independent special /limited diet	Ind. but liquids /special preps.	Manages with help	Needs feeding
6	SLEEPING	Good nights	Interrupted nights	Poor nights	Awake at night /asleep by day	Never asleep /always asleep
7	TOILET	Independent	Commode at night	Commode day & night	Occasional accidents	Frequent accidents
8	HEADACHES	None	Occasionally	Some of the time	A lot of the time	All of the time
9	HEARING	Satisfactory	Slight impairment	Hard of hearing can lip read	Hard of hearing can't lip read	Totally deaf
10	SIGHT	Satisfactory	Some difficulty	Cannot read	Cannot watch television	Blind or almost
11	HEALTH	Good	Good on the whole	Moderate	Poor	Very poor
12	SAD/WEEPY /DEPRESSED	Not at all	Occasionally	Some of the time	A lot of the time	All of the time
13	WORRY	Not at all	Occasionally	Some of the time	A lot of the time	All of the time
14	CONFUSION	Not at all	Occasionally	Some of the time	A lot of the time	All of the time
15	COMPANIONSHIP	Good	Some, no more required	Some but more required	Little, no more required	Little more required
16	PRESENT HELP	None required	Some needed & provided	Much needed & provided	More required	Much more required
17	CARER(S)	None required	Carer(s) have no difficulty	Carer(s) have some difficulty	Carer(s) under stress	Carer(s) cannot continue
18	HOME/HOUSING	Good	Adequate	Inadequate	Untidy or hazardous	Bad

Completed by: Date:

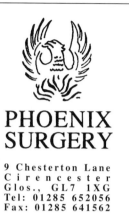

PHOENIX SURGERY

9 Chesterton Lane
Cirencester
Glos., GL7 1XG
Tel: 01285 652056
Fax: 01285 641562

Also at Kemble
& South Cerney

Dear

Your Doctor invites you to make an appointment for an Annual Medical Review, following this visit and completed questionnaire. As this includes a review of your medication and a health check for such things as hearing and sight, it would be very beneficial.

When making your appointment, please tell the receptionist that you wish to have an Annual Medical Review and ask for a double appointment.

Please bring a fresh urine specimen to your appointment.

If you are unable to attend surgery, please ask your Doctor to visit.

Yours sincerely

Hilary Crisp (Mrs)
On behalf of the Doctors, Phoenix Surgery.

Dr H.C.C. Coleridge, Dr D.L. Beales, Dr I.J. Simpson, Dr C.J. Goldie, Dr M.A. Bielenky, Dr R. Sethi

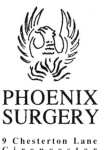

**PHOENIX
SURGERY**

9 Chesterton Lane
Cirencester
Glos., GL7 1XG
Tel: 01285 652056
Fax: 01285 641562

Also at Kemble
& South Cerney

Liz Hicks – Health Visitor/Co-Ordinator
Hilary Crisp Administrative Co-Ordinator
Tel: 01285 659235
STAYWELL 75+ VOLUNTEER VISITING SCHEME

Dear
We should like to introduce you to this successful and well-received scheme which aims to improve our service to older patients in the Practice.

With your permission we should like to ask a trained Volunteer Visitor to contact you during the next few weeks to complete a health questionnaire and to enquire about any day to day difficulties you may be experiencing. The visitor is able to inform you of local services and can act as a link between you and the Practice.

The information you give on every occasion will be treated with the strictest confidence and will be analysed by your doctor, and other health professionals. Any problems that you may have will be followed up. Regular visits may be offered by the volunteer where appropriate.

Each visitor will carry a 'passport card' which you should check with the name at the end of this letter. Please contact Liz Hicks or Hilary Crisp on the above telephone number if you have any queries or do not wish to receive a visitor.

Yours sincerely,

David L. Beales MRCP MRCGP DCH DRCOG

Your visitor will be Mr/Mrs ....
and you will be contacted in the near future.

Dr H.C.C. Coleridge, Dr D.L. Beales, Dr I.J. Simpson, Dr C.J. Goldie, Dr M.A. Bielenky, Dr R. Sethi

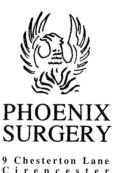

PHOENIX SURGERY

9 Chesterton Lane
Cirencester
Glos., GL7 1XG
Tel: 01285 652056
Fax: 01285 641562

Also at Kemble
& South Cerney

Dear

The enclosed questionnaire is being used by Phoenix practice to help us assess any needs and problems that you might have.

It would be very helpful if you or someone who cares for you could fill it in and return it to the surgery. The information you give will be treated in the strictest confidence and will be analysed by health professionals within the practice.

Our policy is to offer an Annual Medical Review to all patients over 75 years. Please contact the surgery to make an appointment with your doctor, asking for an Annual Medical Review. We should be grateful if you could bring a urine specimen when you come.

Please could you return your questionnaire as soon as possible?

If you have any problems with the form, please telephone Liz Hicks or Hilary Crisp on Cirencester 659235 Monday to Friday between 9 am and 10 am.

Thank you for your co-operation.

Yours sincerely

Mrs E Hicks, Health Visitor for the Elderly
Mrs H Crisp, Staywell 75+ Administrative Co-ordinator

Dr H.C.C. Coleridge, Dr D.L. Beales, Dr I.J. Simpson, Dr C.J. Goldie, Dr M.A. Bielenky, Dr R. Sethi

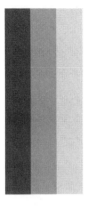

Further information

England

ABBEYFIELDS SOCIETY
53 Victoria Street
St Albans
Herts AL1 3UW
Tel: 01727 857536.

ACCESS COMMITTEE FOR ENGLAND
12 City Forum
250 City Road
London EC1V 8AF
Tel: 0171 250 0008.

ACROSS TRUST
Bridge House
70–72 Bridge Road
East Molesley
Surrey KT8 9HF
Tel: 0181 783 1355.

ACTION FOR BENEFITS, D.S.S.
15 Park Lane
Leeds
West Yorkshire LS1 2SJ
Tel: 0113 245 3353.

ACTION FOR DYSPHASIC ADULTS
1 Royal Street
London SE1 7LL
Tel: 0171 261 9572.

ADVOCACY, CITIZEN INFORMATION AND
   TRAINING
Unit 2K, Leroy House
436 Essex Road
London N1 3QP
Tel: 0171 359 8289.

AGE AND DISABILITY (BT)
Postpoint 207
Exbridge House
Commercial Road
Exeter, Devon EX2 4BB
Call 150.

AGE CONCERN ENGLAND
Astral House
1268 London Road
London SW16 4ER
Tel: 0181 679800. A centre of policy, research,
information and social advocacy on all subjects
regarding the welfare of elderly people.

AGEING, THE CENTRE FOR POLICY ON
25–31 Ironmongers Row
London EC1V 3QP
Tel: 0171 253 1787.

ALZHEIMER'S DISEASE SOCIETY
Gordon House
10 Greencroft Place
London SW1P 1PH
Tel: 0171 306 0606.

ARTHRITIS CARE
18 Stephenson Way
London NW1 2HD
Tel: 0171 916 1500 Hotline: 0800 289170.

ARTHRITIS AND RHEUMATISM COUNCIL
  FOR RESEARCH
Copeman House
St Mary's Court
Chesterfield
Derbyshire S41 7TD
Tel: 01242 558003.

ALCOHOLICS ANONYMOUS
PO Box 1, Stonebow House
Stonebow
York YO1 2NJ
Tel: 01904 644026.

BACKPAIN, NATIONAL ASSOCIATION
16 Elm Tree Road
Teddington
Middlesex TW11 8ST
Tel: 0181 977 5474.

BENEVOLENT ASSOCIATION, NATIONAL
61 Bayswater Road
London WC2 3PG
Tel: 0171 723 0021.

BENEVOLENT FUND FOR THE AGED,
  NATIONAL
1 Leslie Grove Place
Croydon CR0 6TJ
Tel: 0181 688 6655.

BLIND, GENERAL WELFARE OF THE
GWB Products
37–55 Ashburton Grove
London N7 7DW
Tel: 0171 609 0206.

BLIND, GUIDE DOGS FOR THE
Hillfields
Burghfield Common
Reading RG7 37G
Tel: 01734 835555.

BLIND, NATIONAL LIBRARY FOR THE
Cromwell Road
Bredbury
Cheshire SK6 2SG
Tel: 0161 491 0217.

BLIND, ROYAL NATIONAL INSTITUTE
  FOR THE
224–228 Great Portland Street
London W1N 6AA
Tel: 0171 388 1266.

BLIND FUND, TELEPHONES FOR THE
7 Huntersfield Close
Reigate
Surrey RH2 0DX
Tel: 01737 248032.

BLIND FUND, BRITISH WIRELESS
  FOR THE
Gabriel House
34 New Road
Chatham
Kent ME4 4QR
Tel: 01634 832501.

BRITISH ASSOCIATION FOR SERVICE TO THE
  ELDERLY (BASE)
Guildford Institute of University of Surrey
Ward Street
Guildford
Surrey GU1 4LH
Tel: 01483 451036. Advocates the multi-
disciplinary approach to caring for elderly
people and runs courses.

BRITISH DIABETIC ASSOCIATION
10 Queen Anne Street
London W1M 0BD
Tel: 0171 323 1531. Offers advice on diet, aids
and holidays.

BRITISH GERIATRICS SOCIETY
1 St Andrew's Place
London NW1 4LB
Tel: 0171 935 4004.

BRITISH LEGION, THE ROYAL
48 Pall Mall
London SW1Y 5JY
Tel: 0171 930 8131 Hotline: 0345 725725.

BRITISH RED CROSS SOCIETY
9 Grovesnor Square
London SW1X 7EJ
Tel: 0171 235 5454.

CANCER CARE SOCIETY
21 Zetland Road
Redland
Bristol BS6 7AH
Tel: 0117 942 7419.

CANCER HELP CENTRE
Grove House
Cornwallis Grove
Bristol BS8 4PG
Tel: 0117 973 0500.

CANCER RELIEF/MACMILLAN FUND
Anchor House
15–19 Britten Street
London SW3 3TZ
Tel: 0171 351 7811.

CANCER UNITED PATIENTS, BRITISH
ASSOCIATION OF
3 Bath Place
Rivington Street
London EC2A 3JR
Tel: 0800 181199.

CARERS NATIONAL ASSOCIATION
20–25 Glasshouse Yard
London EC1A 4JS
Tel: 0171 490 8818. Helps carers who care for
elderly or disabled dependants.

CHARITY COMMISSION
St Albans House
57 Haymarket
London SW1Y 4QX
Tel: 0171 210 4556.

CITIZENS' ADVICE BUREAUX, NATIONAL
ASSOCIATION OF
115–123 Pentonville Road
London N1 9LZ
Tel: 0171 833 2181.

COLOSTOMY ASSOCIATION, BRITISH
15 Station Road
Reading
Berkshire RG1 1LG
Tel: 01734 391537.

COMMUNITY HEALTH COUNCILS IN
ENGLAND AND WALES, ASSOCIATION OF
30 Drayton Park
London N5 1PB
Tel: 0171 609 8405.

CONSUMERS' ASSOCIATION
PO Box 44
Hertford SG14 1SH
Tel: 0645 123580.

CONTACT
15 Henrietta Street
Covent Garden
London WC2 8QH
Tel: 0171 240 0630.

COUNSEL AND CARE FOR THE ELDERLY
Twyman House
16 Bonny Street
London NW1 9LR
Tel: 0171 485 1566. Provides a free advisory
service to elderly people on any matter of
concern. Information on nursing and residential
care homes.

CROSSROAD CARE ATTENDANT SCHEMES,
ASSOCIATION OF
10 Regent Place
Rugby
Warwickshire CV21 2PN
Tel: 01788 573653. Sends in trained care
attendants to look after the sick and give carers
a break.

CRUSE-BEREAVEMENT CARE
Cruse House
126 Sheen Road
Richmond TW9 1UR
Tel: 0181 332 7227. Offers counselling, advice
and opportunities for social contact for all
widows and widowers.

DEAF ASSOCIATION, THE BRITISH
38 Victoria Place
Carlisle
Cumbria CA1 1HU
Tel: 01228 48844.

DEAF/BLIND HELPERS LEAGUE, NATIONAL
18 Rainbow Court
Paston Ridings
Peterborough PE4 6UP
Tel: 01733 573511.

DEPARTMENT OF HEALTH
Richmond House
79 Whitehall
London SW1A 2NS
Tel: 0171 210 3000.

DEPRESSION ALLIANCE
The Chandlery
50 Westminster Bridge Road
London SE1 7PY
Tel: 0171 721 7672.

DIAL UK
Park Lodge
St Catherines Hospital
Doncaster
South Yorkshire DN4 8QN
Tel: 01302 310123. Telephone information
service for the disabled.

DIEL
Room 1–1
50 Ludgate Hill
London EC4M 7JJ
Tel: 0171 634 8770. Provides independent
bridge between disabled and elderly and
telecommunications industry.

DISABILITY ALLIANCE
Universal House
88–94 Wentworth Street
London E1 7SA
Tel: 0171 247 8763.

DISABLED LIVING FOUNDATION
380–384 Harrow Road
London W9 2HU
Tel: 0171 289 6111.

EPILEPSY, BRITISH ASSOCIATION FOR
Anstey House
40 Hannover Square
Leeds LS3 1BE
Tel: 0800 309030.

EXTEND
22 Maltings Drive
Wheathampstead
Herts AL4 8QJ
Tel: 01582 832760.

FRIENDS OF ELDERLY AND GENTLEFOLKS
42 Ebury Street
London SW1 0LZ
Tel: 0171 730 8263.

GRACE
35 Walnut Tree Close
Guildford
Surrey GU1 4UL
Tel: 01483 304354.

HEALTH EDUCATION AUTHORITY
Hamilton House
Mabledon Place
London WC1H 9TX
Tel: 0171 383 3833.

HEALTH VISITORS' ASSOCIATION
50 Southwark Street
London SE1 1UN
Tel: 0171 717 4000.

HEARING AID COUNCIL
Witan Court
305 Upper Fourth Street
Central Milton Keynes MK9 1EH
Tel: 01908 235700.

HEARING CONCERN
7–11 Armstrong Road
London W3 7JL
Tel: 0181 743 1110.

HELP THE AGED
16–18 St James' Walk
London EC1R 0BE
Senior Line: 0800 289 404.

INTERNATIONAL GLAUCOMA ASSOCIATION
c/o King's College Hospital
Denmark Hill
London SE5 9RS
Tel: 0171 737 3265.

INVALIDS AT HOME TRUST
17 Lapstone Gardens
Harrow
Middlesex HA3 0EB
Tel: 0181 907 1706.

MARIE CURIE MEMORIAL FOUNDATION
28 Belgrave Square
London SW1 1QG
Tel: 0171 235 3325.

MENTAL AFTERCARE ASSOCIATION (MACA)
Bainbridge House
Bainbridge Street
London WC1A 1HP
Tel: 0171 436 6194.

MENTAL HEALTH FOUNDATION
37 Mortimer Street
London W1N 8JU
Tel: 0171 580 0145.

MIND–THE MENTAL HEALTH CHARITY
Granta House
15–19 Broadway
London E15 4BQ
Tel: 0181 522 1728.

NATIONAL ASSOCIATION OF WIDOWS
54–57 Allison Street
Digbeth
Birmingham B5 5TH
Tel: 0121 643 8348. Offers comfort, support
and help to all widows, many of whom are
elderly.

NATIONAL COUNCIL FOR VOLUNTARY
    ORGANIZATIONS (NCVO)
Regent's Wharf
8 All Saints Street
London N1 9RL
Tel: 0171 713 6161.

NATIONAL FEDERATION OF HOUSING
    ASSOCIATIONS
175 Gray's Inn Road
London WC1X 8UP
Tel: 0171 278 6571.

OPEN UNIVERSITY
Portland Tower
Portland Street
Manchester M1 3LD
Tel: 0161 245 3300.

OSTEOPOROSIS SOCIETY, NATIONAL
National Osteoporosis Secretary
PO Box 10
Bath BA3 3YB
Tel: 01761 471771.

PARKINSON'S DISEASE SOCIETY
22 Upper Woburn Place
London WC1H 0RA
Tel: 0171 383 3513.

PARTIALLY SIGHTED SOCIETY
PO Box 322
Doncaster DN1 2XA
Tel: 01302 323132.

PRE-RETIREMENT ASSOCIATION
24 Frederick Sanger Road
Surrey Research Park
Guildford GU5 5YD
Tel: 01483 301170.

QUIT
Victory House
170 Tottenham Court Road
London WC1 0HA
Tel: 0171 388 5775. The national society of
non-smokers.

REACH
Bear Wharf
27 Bankside
London SE1 9ET
Tel: 0171 928 0452.

ROYAL COLLEGE OF NURSING
20 Cavendish Square
London W1M 0AB
Tel: 0171 872 0840.

ROYAL ASSOCIATION FOR DISABILITY AND
    REHABILITATION
12 City Forum
250 City Road
London EC1V 8AF
Tel: 0171 250 3222.

ROYAL NATIONAL INSTITUTE FOR THE DEAF
19–23 Featherstone Street
London EC1Y 8SL
Tel: 0171 296 8001.

ROYAL SOCIETY FOR THE PREVENTION OF
    ACCIDENTS
Edgbaston Park
353 Bristol Road
Birmingham B5 7SW
Tel: 0121 248 2000.

RUKBA
6 Avonmore Road
London W14 8RL
Tel: 0171 602 6274.

SAGA
Freepost 814
Middlesburg Square
Folkestone
Kent CT20 1AZ
Tel: 0800 300 600.

SAMARITANS
10 The Grove
Slough
Berks SL1 1SN
Tel: 01753 532713.

SEXUAL AND PERSONAL RELATIONSHIPS OF
  PEOPLE WITH A DISABILITY
286 Camden Road
London N7 0BJ
Tel: 0171 607 8851. Provides information and
advice on problems in sex and personal
relationships which disability can cause.

STROKE ASSOCIATION
CHSA House
Whitecross Street
London EC1Y 8JJ
Tel: 0171 490 7999.

THE NATIONAL LISTENING LIBRARY
12 Lant Street
London SE1 1BR
Tel: 0171 407 9417.

TINNITUS, BRITISH ASSOCIATION FOR
Room 6
14–18 West Bar Green
Sheffield
South Yorkshire S1 2DA
Tel: 0114 279 6600.

TRISCOPE
The Courtyard
Evelyn Road
London W4 5JL
Tel: 0181 994 9294. Provides nationwide travel
and transport, information and advice services
for disabled and older people, e.g. planning trips,
accessible toilets, mini-bus or wheelchair hire.

UNIVERSITY OF THE THIRD AGE
26 Harrison Street
London WC1H 8JG
Tel: 0171 837 8838.

WOMAN'S ROYAL VOLUNTARY SERVICE
234–244 Stockwell Road
London SW9 9SP
Tel: 0171 416 0146.

WORKER'S EDUCATIONAL ASSOCIATION
Temple House
17 Victoria Park Square
London E2 9PB
Tel: 0181 983 1515. Provides a range of
courses for persons of all age groups. Caters
specifically for older people where there is a
local demand.

Northern Ireland

AGE CONCERN
3 Lower Crescent
Belfast BT7 1NR
Tel: 01232 245729.

ALZHEIMER'S DISEASE SOCIETY
403 Lisburn Road
Belfast BT9 7EW
Tel: 01232 664100.

ARTHRITIS CARE
13 New Forge Lane
Belfast BT9 5NW
Tel: 01232 669882.

CHEST, HEART & STROKE ASSOCIATION
21 Dublin Road
Belfast BT2 7FJ
Tel: 01232 320184.

CROSSROADS CARE ATTENDANT SCHEME
7 Regent Street
Newtownards
County Down BT23 4AB
Tel: 01247 814455.

EXTRACARE FOR ELDERLY PEOPLE
11a Wellington Park
Belfast BT9 6DJ
Tel: 01232 683273.

NATIONAL ASSOCIATION
  OF CARERS
113 University Street
Belfast BT7 1HB
Tel: 01232 439843.

NORTHERN IRELAND SERVICE
  BUREAU (RNIB)
40 Linenhall Street
Belfast BT2 8BG
Tel: 01232 329 1373.

Scotland

AGE CONCERN
113 Rose Street
Edinburgh EH2 3DT
Tel: 0131 220 3345.

ALZHEIMER SCOTLAND ACTION
    ON DEMENTIA
8 Hill Street
Edinburgh EH2 3JZ
Tel: 0131 225 1453.

BENEFITS AGENCY
Central Office for Scotland
Argyle House
3 Lady Lawson Street
Edinburgh EH3 9SH
Tel: 0131 222 5227.

CHEST, HEART & STROKE ASSOCIATION
65 North Castle Street
Edinburgh EH2 3LT
Tel: 0131 225 6963.

CITIZENS' ADVICE SCOTLAND
26 George Square
Edinburgh EH8 9LD
Tel: 0131 667 0156.

CROSSROADS CARE ATTENDANT SCHEME
24 St George Square
Glasgow G2 1EG
Tel: 0141 226 3793.

DISABILITY SCOTLAND
Princes House
5 Shandwick Place
Edinburgh EH2 4RG
Tel: 0131 229 8632.

HEALTH EDUCATION BOARD FOR
    SCOTLAND
Woodburn House
Canaan Lane
Edinburgh EH10 4SG
Tel: 0131 447 8044.

RED CROSS SOCIETY
Alexandra House
204 Bath Street
Glasgow G2 4HL
Tel: 0141 332 9591.

RNIB SCOTLAND
10 Magdala Crescent
Edinburgh EH12 5BE
Tel: 0131 313 1498.

THE ROYAL BRITISH LEGION
    SCOTLAND
Newhaigh House
Logie Green Road
Edinburgh EH7 4HR
Tel: 0131 557 2782.

SCOTTISH SENSORY CENTRE
Holyrood Road
Edinburgh EH8 8AQ
Tel: 0131 558 6501.

SCOTTISH TRUST FOR THE PHYSICALLY
    DISABLED
894 Shettleston Road
Glasgow G32 7XN
Tel: 0141 764 0630.

VOLUNTARY ORGANIZATION, SCOTTISH
    COUNCIL FOR THE
18–19 Claremont Crescent
Edinburgh EH7 4QD
Tel: 0131 556 3882.

Wales

DISABILITY WALES
Llws lfor Crescent Road
Caerphilly CF83 1XL
Tel: 01222 887325.

WALES COUNCIL FOR THE DEAF
Glenview House
Courthouse Street
Pontypridd CF37 1JY
Tel: 01443 485687.

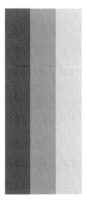

Index

Abbreviated Mental Test
    (AMT) 92, 109–10
abuse 18
accidents 96
acetylcholine 4
Activities of Daily Living (ADL) 109–10, 115,
    116, 169–71
adaptations for daily living 125
advance statements regarding medical treatment
    131–2, 139
adverse drug reactions (ADR) 67–8
aerobic capacity 98–9
Age Concern 125
ageing process 1–2, 7
  advances in treatments 5
  homeostasis 5
  keeping fit 99
  mechanisms or theories 5–7
  physiological changes 2–5
agency 128
agnosia 62
aids for daily living 119, 121, 125
alarm systems 126
albumin 68
alcohol
  congestive heart failure 23
  dementia 58
  ethnic minority groups 143
  falls 49
  health promotion 97
  and nutrition 75
  osteoporosis 40
  tremor 42
alpha-adrenergic blockers 32, 34
alpha-blockers 34
Alzheimer's disease 4
  behavioural problems 61
  diagnosis 59
  presentation 58

Alzheimer's Disease Society 60
amiodarone 22–3, 48
amitriptyline 36
anaemia 18
anhedonia 63
angiotensin converting enzyme (ACE) inhibitors
  21, 22
angiotensin-receptor blockers 21
anterior pituitary hormone secretion 5
anti-cholinergic drugs 34, 41
anticipatory community care 80
  Bicester screening system 157–67
  historical background 81–3
  limitations of conventional care 80–1
  Phoenix Surgery anticipatory care model
    174–6, 188–90
    Cardiff-Newport questionnaire 177–85
    Staywell surveillance system 186–90
  'screening' studies 83–7
anticonvulsant therapy 74
antioxidants 7
anxiety states 63–4
appointeeship 128
apraxia 62
arterial ulcers 46
arthritis 73
aspirin 20, 23, 48
astigmatism 4
atheroma 4
Attendance Allowance 128
attorneys 60, 128, 134
audit 91, 112
autonomy, respect for 137, 138
azapropazone 36
azathioprine 43

back pain 36, 44
Bangladesh 9
Barthel Index 16, 109–10, 115, 116

basal metabolic rate (BMR) 72, 73
BASDEC self-assessment cards 92
bendrofluazide 22
benign prostatic hyperplasia (BPH) 29
benzhexol 41
benzodiazepines 61, 62, 64
beta-blockers
   bradycardias 49
   congestive heart failure 23
   tachycardia 48
   tremor 42
Bicester screening system 82–3, 157–67
biguanides 74
birth rate 10
bisphosphonates 40
Bland, Tony 140
blindness 25, 128
blood pressure 4, 31, 98
blood vessels 4
bone 2
bradycardias 48–9
brain 4
British Red Cross Society 126
bumetanide 22

calcification, cartilage 2
calcium-channel blockers 48, 49, 143
calcium supplements 40
calorie intake 27
cancer 44, 96
   colorectal 27
   prostate 29–30
capacity 130–1, 138
capsaiah ointment 36
captopril 19, 22
carbon monoxide poisoning 17
cardiac myopathy 21
cardiac rehabilitation 21
Cardiff-Newport questionnaire 174–5,
   177–85
cardiovascular system
   ageing process 3–4
   disturbances in cardiac rhythm 48–9
   exercise benefits 100
   see also heart disease
Care and Repair Ltd 127
carers 123, 152–3
   changing attitudes 153–4
   code 155
   community nursing 105–6
   dementia 60–1, 62
   ethical issues 139
   planning with 154

primary health care 154–5
   support 126, 153
Carers (Recognition and Services) Act (1995)
   105–6, 123, 153
cartilage 2–3
catalases 7
catheter infections and blockage 29
cerebellum 4
cerebral cortex 4
chemical abuse 18
chlorpromazine 28, 42
cholecalciferol 27
cigarette smoking 40, 96–7
clock-face test 92–3
codeine 36
codeine phosphate 35
coeliac disease 26
colchicine 36
colitis 27
colon 73
colorectal cancer 27
Committee on Medical Aspects of Food Policy
   (COMA) 73
communication 105, 154
Community Dietetics Service 75
community health services 145
community nursing 102–3, 106–7
   case history 106
   patient as co-worker 105–6
   primary health care team 103–4
   professions allied to medicine 105
   rehabilitation 119
   teamwork 104–5
community occupational therapists 119
community pharmacists 69
community physiotherapists 119
community psychiatric nurses (CPNs) 104–5
community transport 126
compliance problems 67–8
compulsory detention and treatment
   132–4
computer systems 90
confidentiality 105
congestive heart failure (CHF) 21–3
conjunctivitis 18
connective tissues 2, 4
consent to treatment 131, 133, 139
constipation 27
continuing care *see* institutional care
cornea 4
coronary artery disease 20
   ageing process 3–4
   ethnic minority groups 143

exercise 101
  Health of the Nation 96
corticosteroids 18, 36, 43
costal cartilage 2
counselling 96–7, 126
Court of Protection 128
C-reactive protein (CRP) 37
creatinine, serum 28–9
Crossroads schemes 126
curatory 134–5
cytoprotection 36

day care 126, 127
day hospitals 120
deafness 25, 128
delirium 25, 57–8
  behavioural problems 61
  urinary incontinence 32
dementia 55–62
  abbreviated mental test and clock-face test
      92–3
  community psychiatric nursing 104
  and nutrition 74
demography of old age 9, 14
  ethnic minority groups 141
  late-age mortality trends and population
      predictions 11–12
  morbidity in later life 12–13
  perceptions and realities of ageing 9–10
  regional variations 13–14
dentures 26, 73
dependency 75, 110
depression 61, 62–3, 104
detrusor-sphincter-dyssynergia 32, 34
dexamethasone 43
diabetes mellitus 37–9
  ethnic minority groups 143–4
  feet 25
  hypothermia 28
diabetic neuropathy 32
diabetic retinopathy 25
dial-a-ride schemes 126
diarrhoea 35
diastolic dysfunction 23
diet see nutrition
dietary reference values (DRVs) 73, 74
digoxin
  bradycardias 49
  congestive heart failure 22
  renal function 29
  tachycardia 48
Diploma in Geriatric Medicine 147–51
disability 114–17, 121–2, 126

see also rehabilitation
Disability Living Allowance 127
disposable soma theory 6
Disposal of Unwanted Medicine and Poison
      (DUMP) campaigns 69
district nurses 104, 106
diuretics 22
dizziness 24–5, 67
DNA 6, 7
domperidone 41
door-to-door transport 126
dopamine 5
driving 60, 126
drug-nutrient interactions 74
Dyazide 22
dyspnoea 21
dysrhythmias 22–3

ears 5, 25
ECHO-cardiography 20, 21, 22, 23
Elderly Accommodation Council 127
e-mail 119
endocrine system 5, 7, 73
end-of-life decisions 139–40
Enduring Power of Attorney (EPA) 60, 128
enemas 35
errors in protein synthesis theory about ageing
      6–7
erythrocyte sedimentation rate (ESR) 37
estimated average requirement (EAR) 73
ethical issues 136–7
  aims of elderly care 137
  capacity 138
  'end-of-life' decisions 139–40
  interface with other agencies 138–9
  resource allocation 140
  risk-taking 137–8
  vulnerability 138
ethnic minority groups 141
  coronary artery disease 143
  demography 141
  diabetes mellitus 143–4
  disease patterns 142–3
  functional ability 144
  hypertension and stroke 143
  osteomalacia 144
  positive discrimination 145–6
  social concerns 141–2
  social services 145
  tuberculosis 144
  use and awareness of services 144–5
euthanasia 131
evolution of ageing 6

exercise
  cardiovascular system 4
  congestive heart failure 21
  health promotion 97, 98–101
  myocardial infarction 21
exertional hypotension 31, 48
extended families 142
extra-pyramidal defects 31, 41
eyes 4–5, 25

faecal incontinence 27, 35
falls 28, 49–51, 112
fat, body 2, 72
feet 25–6
fertility 9–10, 11–12
fibrocartilage 2
financial issues
  advice and assistance 127–8
  carers 153, 155
  mental disease 60
fitness 98–101
flavoxate 34
fluoride therapy 40
folate deficiency 27
fractures, 2, 40
free-radical theory about ageing 7
Frenchay Activities Index 115
frontal-lobe dementia 58, 63
frusemide 22
fundholding GPs 70, 104–5, 119

gait apraxias 31
gastric ulcers 26
gastrointestinal tract 26–7, 72–3
gene expression 7
General Practitioners Charter (1966) 103
genitourinary system 28–9
genome-based theories about ageing 6
gentamicin 29
Geriatric Depression Scale (GDS) 55, 57, 92
geriatric health visitor (GHV) 92
Geriatric Medicine Diploma 147–51
ghee 143
giant cell arteritis (GCA) 42–3
giardiasis 26
giddiness 25
glaucoma 19, 25
glibenclamide 38
glomerular filtration rate (GFR) 28–9
glutathione 7
glutathione reductase 7
gluten enteropathy 26
gout 36–7

Griffiths, Sir Roy 123
growth hormone (GH) 3, 5
guardianship 133
gut ischaemia 27

H2 36
hallucinations 61
haloperidol 61
handicap 114–17
Health of the Nation 96
health promotion 95–6
  counselling 96–7
  immunization 98
  keeping fit 98–101
  screening 97–8
health visitors 104
hearing 5, 25, 128
hearing aids 111, 128
heart disease
  clinical diagnosis of heart failure 21–2
  congestive cardiac failure 21, 22–3
  hypertension 18–20
  myocardial infarction 20–1
heart failure 21–3
heparin 20–1
herpes simplex 18
herpes zoster 18
holiday heart 23
holidays 127
home-based rehabilitation 118, 120–1
Home Energy Efficiency Scheme (HEES)
    127
home-help services 125
homeostasis 1, 5
hormone replacement therapy 40
hospital-at-home schemes 118
household size, ethnic minority groups
    142
housing services 127
hypercalcaemia 37
hypernatraemia 37
hypertension 18–20, 143
hyperthyroidism 39, 73
hypnotics 49
hypoglycaemia 28, 38
hypokalaemia 22
hypomania 63
hyponatraemia 37
hypotension 31, 47–8
hypothalamic lesions 39
hypothalamus 5
hypothermia 17, 28
hypothyroidism 39, 73

ibuprofen 36
idiopathic Parkinson's disease (IPD) 41
imipramine 34, 36
immobility 30–1, 32
immune system 7
immunization 98
immunosuppression 18
impaired glucose tolerance 38
impairment 114–17
Income Support 128
incontinence
    faecal 27, 35
    urinary 29, 31–5, 129
Independent Living Fund 127
infant mortality 11, 14
infections 73, 112
inflammatory arthropathies 36–7
influenza vaccine 98, 112
information systems 92
institutional care 108–9
    assessment 109–10
    care planning 110–11
    future possibilities 112–13
    prescribing 69–70
    quality assurance 112
    risk management 112
    routine surveillance 111–12
    systematized care 111
intervertebral discs 2–3
invalid care allowance 128
iron-deficiency anaemia 18
ischaemic ulcers 46

justice 137

lactulose 36
language, ethnic minority groups 142
large bowel 27
laundry services 129
laxatives 35, 36
l-dopa 41, 42
lean-body mass 72
legal issues 60, 127–8, 130
    advance statements regarding medical
        treatment 131–2
    capacity 130–1
    compulsory detention and treatment 132–4
    consent to medical treatment 131
    medical treatment at end of life 132
    property management 134–5
lens 4
life expectancy 9, 12, 14
lipofuscin 4

liver function 68
living arrangements 60
'Living Wills' 131–2, 139
local authority service provision 124–5
lofepramine 63
longevity 1
long-sightedness 4
long-term medication 67
lower-limb skin ulceration 46
lowest reference nutrient intake (LRNI) 73
luncheon clubs 125

Madopar 41
malabsorption 26
malignant neuroleptic syndrome 42
malnutrition 18
manic-depressive illness 63
Manrex 69
maximal oxygen uptake 99
McIntosh over 75s assessment questionnaire
    168–73
meals provision 125
medical assessment questionnaire 172
memory 4, 58, 59
men
    cardiovascular system 3
    coronary artery disease 20
    mortality 11, 14
    osteoporosis 2, 40
    urinary incontinence 31, 34
menopause 2, 40
mental disease, presentation and management
    54–5, 96
    see also named diseases
Mental Health Act (1983) 55, 64, 132–3
Mental Heath Review Tribunals (MHRT) 133
mental status questionnaire 172–3
metabolic disorders 37
metformin 74
Methotrexate 43
middle-ear disease 67
Mini-Mental State Examination (MMSE) 55,
    56, 59
misoprostal 36
moclobemide 63
morbidity in later life 12–13
morphine sulphate 36
mortality, late-age 11–12, 14
motivation, exercise 101
mouth 26, 72–3
movement disorders 41–2
multi-disciplinary team, rehabilitation 119
multiple myeloma 18, 37

muscle 3, 5, 99
musculoskeletal system 2–3, 35–6
  exercise 100
  and nutrition 73
myocardial infarction 20–1, 143
myositis 44

National Assistance Act (1948) 133–4
National Health Service and Community Care
    Act (1990) 123, 124
nervous system 4
neuroendocrine factors 5
neuroendocrine system 7
neurofibrillary tangle (NFT) 4
neurogenic dysphagia 74
neuroleptics 42, 61
neurotransmitters 4, 5
nocturnal paroxysms 23
nocturnal retinal ischaemia 19
Nomad 69
non-genomic theories about ageing 6–7
non-insulin-dependent diabetes mellitus
    (NIDDM) 37–8, 143–4
non-steroidal anti-inflammatory drugs (NSAIDs)
    26, 36, 37
noradrenaline 4, 5
Norton Scale of pressure-sore risk 45
Nottingham Extended ADL Scale 115
nurses
  prescribing 69, 70
  screening 92–3, 158
  see also community nursing
nursing homes see institutional care
nutrition 72
  cardiovascular system 4
  case presentation 77–8
  deficiencies 26–7
  extrinsic factors 74–5
  improvements 77
  intrinsic factors 72–3
  meals provision 125
  osteoporosis 40
  pathological factors 73–4
  risk recognition, poor nutritional status 75–6

occupational therapy 105, 118, 119, 121
oesophagus 26
oestrogen deficiency 29
orange-badge scheme 126
origins of community care 123
orthostatic hypotension 19, 47–8
osteoarthritis 99
osteoarthrosis 35–6

osteomalacia 26–7, 144
osteoporosis 2, 40–1
overgrowth, bacterial 26
over-the-counter (OTC) medication 68–9

pacemakers 49
'pacemaker' theories about ageing 7
pan-hypopituitaryism 39
paracetamol 36
paranoia 61, 64
Parkinson's disease 41–2
  activity levels 99
  behavioural problems 61
  institutional care 112
partially sighted people 128–9
peroxidases 7
persistent vegetative state 140
pharmacists, community 69
pharmacodynamics 68
pharmacokinetics 68
Phenobarbitone 74
phenothiazine 42
phenytoin 74
Phoenix Surgery anticipatory care model 174–6
  Cardiff-Newport questionnaire 177–85
  Staywell surveillance system 186–90
physical abuse 18
physical disease, presentation and management
    15–18
  see also named diseases
physiological changes, ageing process 2–5
physiotherapy 118, 119
primozide 64
pituitary dysfunction 39–40
pituitary hormone secretion 5
planning
  with carers 154
  institutional care 110–11
podiatry 105
poisoning 17
polymyalgia rheumatica (PMR) 42–3
polymyositis 42
polypharmacy 66, 67, 69
potassium 22
Powers of Attorney 128, 134
practice nursing 103–4
prednisolone 37, 43
prescribing 66–7, 70–1
  adverse drug reactions 67–8
  community pharmacist 69
  continuing-care patients 69–70
  nurse prescribing 69
  over-the-counter medication 68–9

Prescription of Medical Products by Nurses Act
    (1992) 69
pressure sores 44–6, 112
primary health care team (PHCT)
    institutional care 111
    nursing 102, 103–4, 105
proctitis 27
progressive supra nuclear palsy 41
property management 134–5
propranolol 42
prostate 29–30
prostate specific antigen (PSA) 30
protein synthesis errors, ageing theory 6–7
proton pump blockers 36
pseudo-gout 36
psychological benefits of exercise 100
public transport 126
Purkinje neurones 4
pyrophosphate-arthropathy 36

quality assurance, institutional care 112
questionnaires
    Cardiff-Newport 174–5, 177–85
    McIntosh over 75s assessment 168–73
    screening and socio-medical assessment
        90, 91
    Winchester 187

race 141
rate of living theory about ageing 6
receivership 134–5
recommended nutritional intake 73
records 105, 106
recreation facilities 127
recurrent urinary infection 29
red blood cells (RBCs) 7
reference nutrient intake (RNI) 73
regional variations, demography 13–14
Registered Homes Act (1984) 70
rehabilitation 117–18
    aids for daily living 121–2
    community services 120–1
    goals 119–20
    multi-disciplinary team 119
renal angioplasty 19
renal function 28–9
    ageing process 72
    hypertension 19
    pharmacokinetics 68
resident assessment protocols (RAPs) 112–13
residential care see institutional care
resource allocation 140
respite care 126, 153

retina 4, 5
rheumatoid arthritis 36–7
risk management, institutional care 112
risk-taking, ethical issues 137–8
risperidone 64
routine surveillance, institutional care 111–12
Rutherglen Experiment 81

safety during exercise 100–1
salt 143
screening 81–7, 157–67
    health promotion 97–8
    practical organization 89–94
scurvy 27
sectioning of patients 133
sedation 69
self-harm, deliberate 17
senile plaques 4
Sheldon, Joseph 114
sheltered housing 127
Shy Drager Syndrome 41
sick euthyroid syndrome 40
Sinemet 41
sitting services 126
skin 2, 5, 46
sleep disturbances 61
smell, sense of 5, 72
smoking 40, 96–7
social deprivation, ethnic minority groups
        141–2
social facilities 127
Social Fund 127
social isolation 75
Social Security benefits 127, 128
social services
    disability assessment 117
    ethnic minority groups 145
    institutional care 108
    rehabilitation 119, 121
    screening and socio-medical assessment 91,
        92
socio-medical assessment 89–94
sodium valproate 42
sotalol 48
spondylosis 36
'Staying Put' 127
Staywell surveillance system 175–6, 186–90
Steele Richardson Syndrome 41
stomach 26, 73
stroke 23–4
    activity levels 99
    ethnic minority groups 143
    Health of the Nation 96

suicide 62
sulphonylurea 38
superoxide dismutase 7
support services
    carers 126, 153, 155
    mental disease 60–1
surveillance
    institutional care 111–12
    Staywell system 175–6, 186–90
suspicion 61
swallowing difficulties 26
syncope 46–7
systematized institutional care 111
systemic lupus erythematosus (SLE) 36, 44
systolic hypertension 19

tachy-arrhythmias 48
tachycardia 48
taste, sense of 5, 72
taxi card schemes 126
teamwork, community nursing 105
telephones 119, 128
temperature, body 5
tetanus toxoid 98
tetrabenazine 42
therapeutic diets 75
thiazides 22, 143
thioridazine 42, 61, 64
third party mandates 128
thrombo-embolic disease 23
thrombolysis 21
thyroid disorders 39
tolbutamide 38
training programmes
    screening and socio-medical assessment
        90–1
    Staywell surveillance system 186
transport 126
trazodone 61, 63
tremor 42
tricyclic antidepressants 34, 61, 63, 74
trifluoperazine 64

trusts 134
tuberculosis 144
tutors-dative system 131
type-A toileting regimen 34
type-B toileting regimen 34

unexplained illness 17–18
urinary incontinence 29, 31–5, 129
urinary infection 29

varicose ulcers 46
vascular Parkinson's disease 41
vasodilators 28
venlafaxine 63
verapamil 23, 48
vertebral collapse 2, 40
vision 4–5, 25
vitamin-C deficiency 27
vitamin-D deficiency 26–7, 40, 144
vitamin E 7
vitreous humor 4–5
vulnerability 138

warfarin 20, 23, 48
waste product theory about ageing 6
water, body 2, 5
wax, ear 25
weight loss 26, 27
weight measurement 112
Winchester Disability Questionnaire
        176, 187
women
    cardiovascular system 3–4
    mortality 12
    osteoporosis 2, 40
    recurrent urinary infection 29
    urinary incontinence 31, 32
Women's Royal Voluntary Service (WRVS)
        125, 126
wound healing 73

xerostomia 26